Dedicated to

SFC Marcus V. Muralles

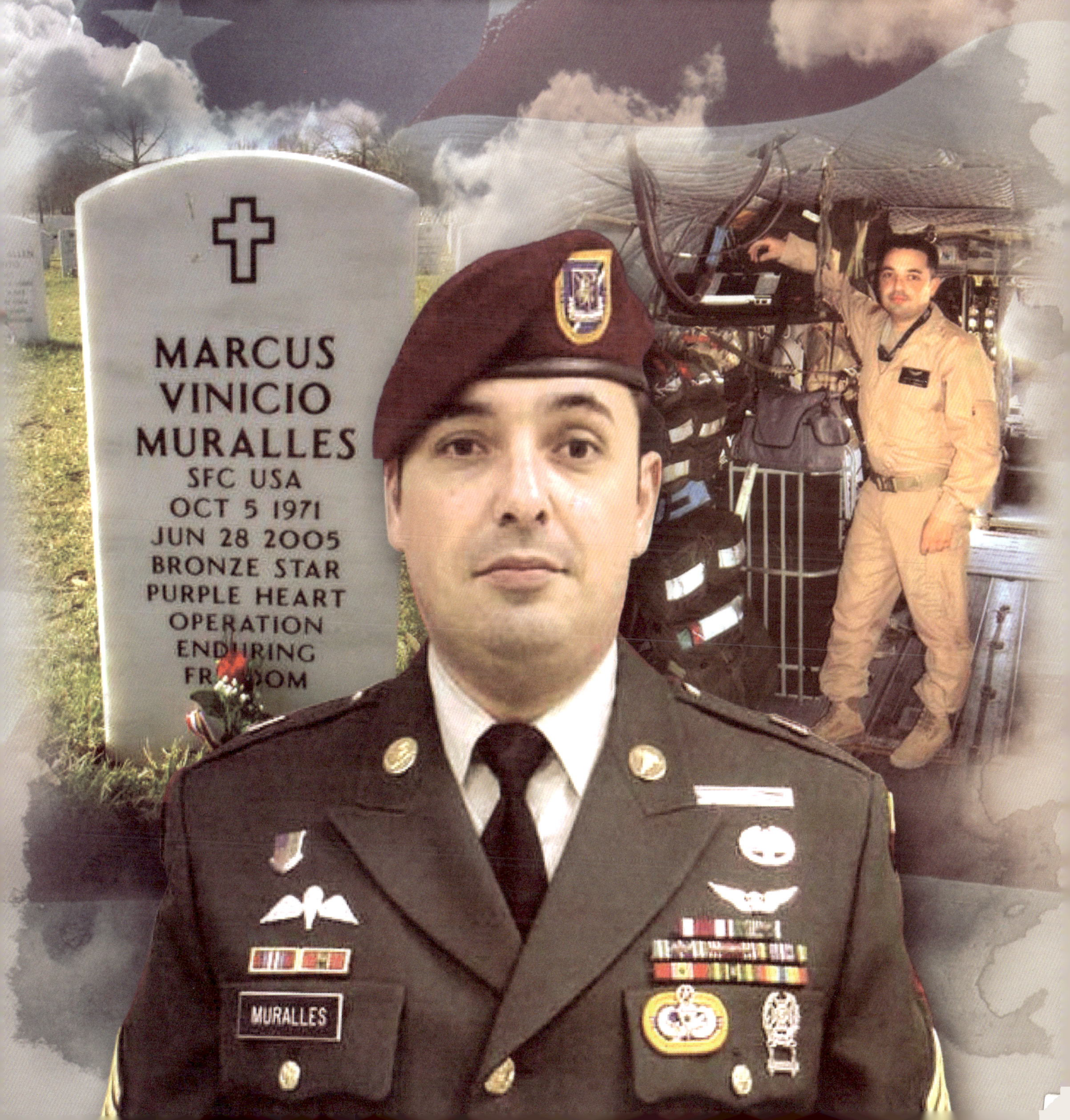

Table of Contents

Visit our website www.immediateactionmedicine.org
ISBN 978-0-615-56313-8

DISCLAIMER

This is document is not to be electronically altered, distributed, copied by any means, or otherwise reproduced without the written permission of the author. This document is protected under U.S. Copyright law and is for reference use only and does not imply any level of medical competency.

The accuracy and completeness cannot be guaranteed. Any medical procedures performed must be done so after individual accreditation and credentialing by local medical authorities. This book is not to be construed as protocol for any medical service.

The author accepts no liability of any medical procedures performed. The Flight Paramedic Certification Guide ©2011 is an independent publication and has not been authorized, sponsored, or otherwise approved by the Board for Critical Care Transport Paramedic Certification (BCCTPC) Inc.

This guide is based on the standards used in the civilian healthcare setting and do not reflect Tactical Combat Casualty Care (TCCC) guidelines in all situations. Use the appropriate guidelines for the environment you find yourself in.

The opinions or assertions herein are the private views of the author and are not to be construed as official or as reflecting the views of the U.S. Army Special Operations Command (USASOC), the Department of the Army (DA), or the Department of Defense (DoD).

How to pass the FP-C Exam

STUDY EFFECTIVELY!

When studying for this exam (or any other exam) remember that your brain can only absorb so much material at a time. Adults learn best through repetition. Read a section, read it again, then move on. Do not read several sections at once until you are doing a final review just before your test. When studying, do so for no more than 50 minutes, and then take a 10 minute break. Most knowledge is retained during the first and last 15 minutes of each study session. This theory has been proven through many studies of adult learning. Studying more does not mean studying effectively. Below are figures for average test scores among a large group of selected test takers. It represents several preparatory courses with varying lengths and test taking strategies.

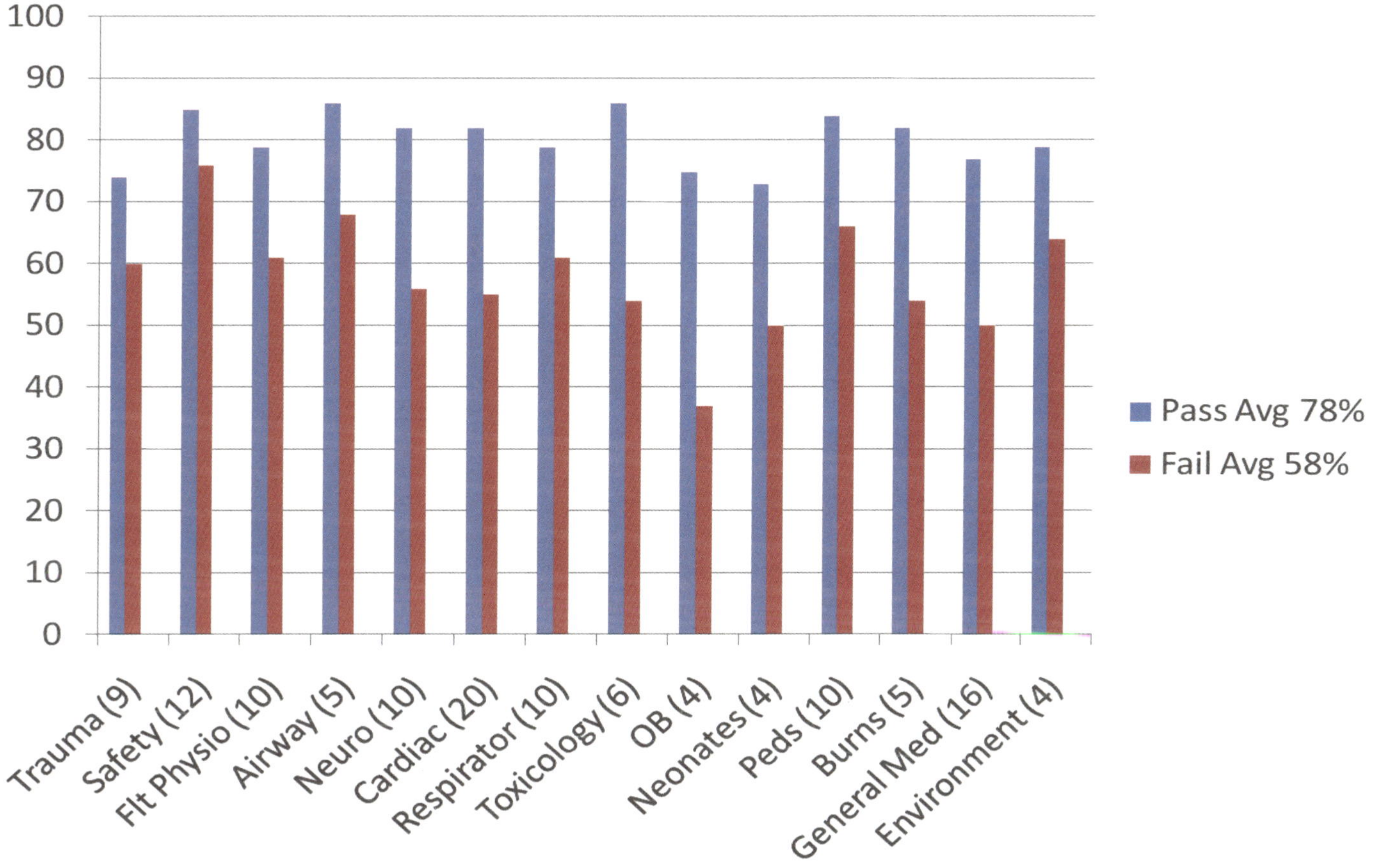

The minimum score required to pass the FP-C exam varies based on the version taken, but is normally around 70-74% (depending on the version of the exam). The FP-C exam does not focus on basic Paramedic skill sets to include ACLS, PALS, etc. This exam is a test of critical care knowledge in the rotary and fixed wing aviation environment. You should take an ACLS and PALS refresher within 6 months of taking an FP-C prep course to refresh your memory. This certification guide covers materials presented in the Immediate Action Medicine, LLC FP-C review course and is based on the exam blueprint written by the BCCTPC.

FP-C Exam Question Blueprint

Trauma Management	9
Aircraft Fundamentals, safety and survival	12
Flight Physiology	10
Advanced Airway Management Techniques	5
Neurological Emergencies	10
Critical Cardiac Patient	20
Respiratory Patient	10
Toxic Exposures	6
Obstetrical Emergencies	4
Neonates	4
Pediatric	10
Burn Patients	5
General Medical Patient	16
Environmental	4
TOTAL	**125**

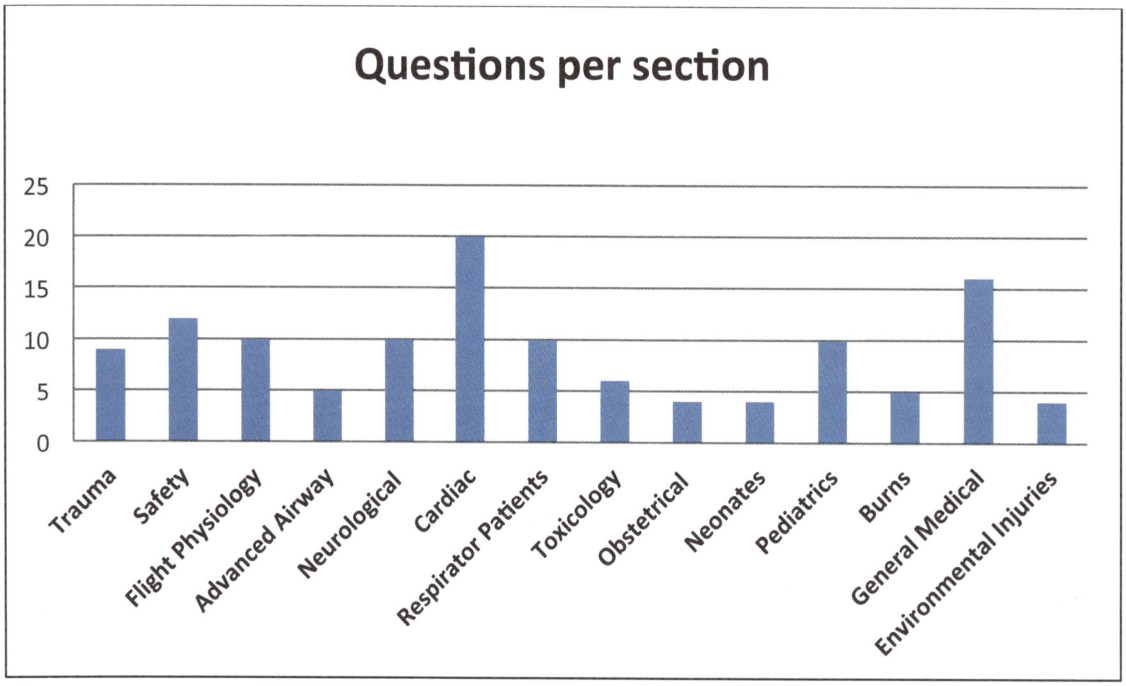

TRAIN AS YOU FIGHT!

Take as many practice questions as possible. You only get faster by running faster, stronger by lifting heavier weights, and better at taking tests by answering more sample test questions. When taking my FP-C course you will take two 135 question tests modeled after the BCCTPC exam. The first one is taken before the class begins, and the last one is taken on the final day of the course. Every day you will take quizzes over each subject to further increase your test-taking skills. My course typically has a high pass average (my first-time pass rate is well above 80%, the national average pass rate is 62%), this is because my students take a lot of practice questions!

If you find that you are unable to do the above mentioned strategies by yourself, find a study partner. BE SELECTIVE! A study group should be small. If you have too many people in your study group it turns into a time to talk about things other than the material. Ask your partner questions without leading them, and if they don't know a particular subject they need to study that subject more. Bottom line-if you don't know a question when your study partner asks, you probably won't know it when the written exam asks the same thing (and your sympathetic nervous system is in high gear).

PASS THE TEST!

When taking this exam you must use a good test taking strategy. There are two ways to take the test; paper or electronic based. If you are more familiar and comfortable with taking paper tests, choose this method. It will require a little more work for you to find a testing site (can be found on the BCCTPC website). You will also have to wait at least 4-6 weeks to get your results if taking a paper exam, whereas when taking the computer-based exam you will have your results instantly. If you are more comfortable with computer based testing, I recommend the online version. This also needs to be coordinated with the BCCTPC office, however it can be done at most major cities with approved testing centers. Contact the BCCTPC and apply for your "AMP Number," which is what you will need to schedule your exam. In the event you do not pass the exam, you must wait 30 days to retake it.

The strategy is simple. Remember that there are NO points for finishing first, and no one impressed when you fail first. Take your time; you have 2 ½ hours to complete the exam. YOU ARE ALLOWED TO USE A SIMPLE CALCULATOR ON THE TEST! Do not look at more than one question at a time, and if taking the computer test only one question will be on the screen at a time. If you are taking the paper test I recommend you take one of the pieces of note paper you are given and cover up the rest of the questions. Cover the entire page, and only expose the question. Read it carefully! Look for words like "always, never, is not, are, false, true, etc." The words that are often overlooked when stressed from test taking and will cause you to miss a question. Once you have read and understand the question, uncover the answers. This is a multiple choice test with 5 possible answers, only one is correct. Choose the most correct answer!

You should use an elimination strategy when taking multiple choice tests. This is done by looking at the possible answers and crossing off the ones you are sure don't answer the question. If there are two similar answers, there is a good chance that one of them is the right one. TAKE A DEEP BREATH AND RELAX. If you have no idea what the answer is, pick "C." This is so you are consistent in your guessing, which will give you a better statistical chance of guessing right.

If you are sure of your answer, go with it. DO NOT CHANGE YOUR ANSWER ONCE YOU CIRCLE IT! The only reason to change answer would be that you are absolutely sure you answered something wrong. You will almost always be wrong if you change your answer, study after study has proven this. Move to the next question.

TAKE BREAKS DURING THE TEST! This can either be done during the test while sitting at your desk or you can leave the room to clear your mind. Recommend getting up from your desk about very 40 -50 questions and taking a five minute break. I have heard the story "I knew the material" more times than I can count (usually when that person is telling me they failed an exam). It is often true that people who know given material fail tests because they are "bad test takers." This is why you need to use a good test taking strategy!

Flight Physiology (10)

GAS LAWS

Boyle's Law "Boyle's = Balloon = Barotrauma"

- The pressure of a gas is inversely proportional to the volume of a gas at a constant temperature

$$P_1V_1 = P_2V_2$$

- Affects ETT cuffs, MAST trousers, Air splints, IV drip rates (increases rate) ↑ air amount
- If the patient has a Pneumocephalus (air inside the cranial vault after trauma, usually from a direct blow, associated with depressed skull fractures) intracranial pressure will increase. ↑ cranial pressure ↑ Altitude

Dalton's Law "Dalton's Gang" — Soft tissue swelling

- Law of Partial Pressures (this is an additive gas law)
- The total pressure of a gas mixture is the sum of the partial pressures of all the gases in the mixture

$$P_T = P_1 + P_2 + P_3 + ... + P_n$$

- Responsible for soft tissue swelling at altitude (uptake of inert gasses into tissue)

Charles' Law "Charging Charles" — Charging O_2 tank ↑ pressure

- At a constant pressure, the volume of gas is directly proportional to the absolute temperature of the gas

$$V_1 / T_1 = V_2 / T_2$$

- Example- When you charge an oxygen tank, the tank gets hot
- This law has very little effect on the human body (we are at a relatively constant temperature)

Gay-Lussac's Law = Colder temp ↓ pressure

- Directly proportional relationship between temperature and pressure

$$P_1 / T_1 = P_2 / T_2$$

- Example- an oxygen cylinder left outside overnight will have a lower pressure reading in the morning due to temperature drop.
- This is the gas law that explains the reason you need to add air to your tires in the winter (colder temps lower pressure)

Graham's Law "Graham's = Grey Matter" ← diffusion of gas through liquid

- Law of Gaseous Diffusion
- "Gas exchange at the cellular level"
  - The rate of diffusion of a gas through a liquid medium is directly related to the solubility of the gas and inversely proportional to the square root of its density
- Limits gas ability to move through liquid
  - Example- *gas bubbles coming out of exposed grey matter when at altitude*

Henry's Law "Henry = Heineken" ← Solubility of gas

- Solubility of gas in liquid
- The quantity of gas dissolved in 1 cm^3 (1 mL) of a liquid is proportional to the partial pressure of the gas in contact with the liquid
- Affects divers, can lead to decompression sickness "the bends"
  - The bends are the most common form of decompression sickness

Gas Law	Pneumonic	Example
Boyle's	Balloon Barotrauma	Air filled medical device expansion/Pneumocephalus/AGE
Dalton's	Dalton's Gang	Soft tissue swelling at altitude
Charles'	Charging Charles	Oxygen tank getting hot when filled
Graham's	Grey Matter	Gas bubbles from exposed grey matter
Henry's	Heineken	Decompression sickness "The Bends"

Decompression Sickness "The Bends"

- Related to Henry's Law
- There are actually 6 different types of DCS , which are too in depth for this guide

Type I– Nitrogen related, painful joints, mottled skin, pruritic (itching)

- Patient may also feel like "ants are crawling on their skin"
- Cutis marmorata- mottled skin, can often look like a sunburn

Type II– Neurologic signs & symptoms, hypovolemic shock

- Ground transport is preferred for all diving injuries/decompression sickness

- Ground transport is preferred for all diving injuries/decompression sickness

Arterial Gas Embolism (AGE)

- Related to Boyle's Law
- Caused breath holding during ascent on a dive, air pushes through the alveoli and enters the skin in the neck/chest
  - Causes a pneumothorax
- Air is forced into blood vessels
  - The air bubble blocks blood vessels, causing ischemia
- Patient presents with stroke-like symptoms (altered mental status, syncope, dizziness)
  - May also have a cough and epistaxis (nosebleed)
- AGE requires immediate hyperbaric treatment!
  - Fly in a pressurized aircraft (fixed wing) or rotary wing <1000ft MSL

Pulmonary Overpressurization

- Related to Boyle's Law
- A syndrome that occurs when "breath holding" compressed air during ascent
  - The greatest pressure differences are just below the surface of the water (≤ 4 ft. depth)
- Causes lung overexpansion and ruptures the alveoli
  - Causes pneumothorax or mediastinal emphysema
- Common in inexperienced divers

Atmosphere Calculations

- Every 33 feet below water 33ft = 1 ATM (atmosphere)
- Sea Level= 1 ATM
- 33 ft. under water = 2 ATM
- 66ft under water = 3 ATM

EXAMPLE: If you pick a patient that was diving at a depth of 33ft, they were exposed to 2 ATM of pressure. This may also be written as 2 atmospheres absolute (2 ATA).

Divers Alert Network

- 24 hour hotline for diving related injuries and questions
- www.diversalertnetwork.org (919) 684-9111

Atmosphere Zones

Physiologic Zone: *Sea Level to 10,000ft MSL*

- Night Vision is decreased beginning at 5,000 ft. MSL

Physiologically Deficient Zone: *10k to 50kft MSL*

- Oxygen or pressurization required to survive at these altitudes
- If in a pressurized cabin and a sudden decompression occurs Time of Useful Consciousness (TUC) is cut in half
  - A sign of compression loss is cooler temperatures in the cabin and windows fogging
  - Normally 90 seconds of useful consciousness at 30,000 ft.
    - If a rapid decompression occurs, TUC is now around 45 sec

Example- If you were in an altitude chamber at 30k ft. and took your oxygen mask off, you would normally have around 90 seconds of consciousness. If you took your mask off and the chamber was rapidly decompressed, you would only have 45 seconds consciousness.

Space Equivalent Zone: *>50kft MSL*

- If you are here, congratulations on becoming an astronaut!

Oxygen Adjustment Calculation

$(FiO_2 x P_1) / P_2$ = FiO2 required for ascent

FiO_2= Fraction of inspired oxygen
P_1= the pressure you are at (on the ground)
P_2= the pressure you are flying to (cruising altitude)

Pressure (P) Values		(torr and mmHg are essentially the same thing)
Sea Level	760 torr or mmHg	(1 ATM)
10k ft. MSL	523 torr or mmHg	
18k ft. MSL	380 torr or mmHg	(1/2 ATM)
63k ft. MSL	0 torr or mmHg	(0 ATM)

Example: You have a patient on a Non-Rebreather Mask at 0.5 FiO_2 and you are at sea level. You will be flying to an altitude with a torr of 500. What will be the oxygen requirement at this pressure?

$$\frac{0.5 \times 760}{500} = 0.76\ FiO2$$ required for ascent (76% oxygen)

Types of Hypoxia

Hypemic "Anemic"

- Reduction in the O_2 carrying capacity of blood
- Anemia, hemorrhage

Histotoxic "Poisoning"

- Limits the use of available oxygen due to poisoning of the cytochrome oxidase system
- Cyanide, Alcohol, Carbon Monoxide (CO), Nitroglycerin, Sodium Nitroprusside (Nipride)

Hypoxic "Not enough Oxygen in the air"

- ↓partial pressure of oxygen at altitude
- Deficiency in alveolar O_2 exchange
- Cardiovascular/ Pneumothorax patients are more susceptible to this type of hypoxia

Stagnant "Blood isn't moving"

- Reduced cardiac output or pooling of blood
- High G forces, cardiogenic shock

Stages of Hypoxia "ICDC"

Stage of Hypoxia	Symptoms
Indifferent	Full reasoning abilities, some loss of night vision
Compensatory	Increased HR, ventilations, slowed judgment
Disturbance	Slurred speech, impaired judgment, "drunk"
Critical	No longer able to physiologically function, death imminent

……. The *Indifferent stage is most important* (because you can still think)

Stressors of Flight

Self Imposed	**Inherent**
Dehydration	Thermal Changes
Exhaustion	↓ Humidity
Alcohol	Gravitational Forces
Tobacco	Fatigue
Hypoglycemia	↓ Partial Pressure of Oxygen
	Barometric Pressure Change
	Noise
	Vibration

G Forces

Gravitational Force	Direction of force	Toleration	Example
G_x	Anterior/Posterior	Best Tolerated	Accelerating in your car
G_z	Vertical		Falling from a roof and landing on your feet
G_y	Lateral	Least tolerated	Being "T-boned" in a car wreck

- G forces can be positive (+) or negative(-)
  - Example: + G_x when a dragster takes off, - G_x when the dragster deploys the parachute

- G forces cause B/P to drop
- People most affected by high G forces
  - On B/P meds (especially Beta Blockers)
  - Dehydrated

Altitude Effects

- A cold, dry, high altitude environment has the greatest negative outcome to your patient
  - Every 1,000 foot increase in elevation causes temperatures to drop 2° C
  - Temperature is inversely proportional to altitude

Barondontalgia (Teeth)

- Occurs on Ascent
- Air trapped in fillings expands due to Boyles law
- *Also referred to as "Aerodontaligia"*

Barotitis (Ears)

- Occurs on Descent
- Air trapped in the middle ear can't vent through the blocked Eustachian Tube (Eustachian Tube Dysfunction)
- *"Ear Block"*

Barosinusitis (Sinuses)

- Can occur on BOTH Ascent and Descent
- Can also cause pain the maxillary teeth (but is not the same as barodontalgia; that occurs only on ascent)
- *"Sinus Block"*

Safety/CAMTS (12)

(Commission for the Accreditation of Medical Transport Systems)

CAMTS is the commission that accredits companies to become medical transport systems. This is similar to a hospital getting accreditation from The Joint Commission (TJC). They also set safety standards, as well as professional conduct standards. Go to www.camts.org for the latest published guidelines.

Air Transport Team Members

- Flight Nurse
- Flight Paramedic
- Respiratory Therapist
- Flight Physician

- The crew mix of any transport system varies by individual company. Most aircraft fly single-pilot, and utilize a Flight Paramedic and a Critical Care Nurse team.

AMRM "Air Medical Resource Management"

- Distributes workload
- "The operational practice of involving ALL members of the flight team (pilot and clinical crew members) in the mission planning, decision making, and mission safety
- Referred to as CRM (Crew Resource Management) in the military

Sterile cockpit

- Only essential communication during all phases of flight except straight and level flight
- Critical phases of flight: Takeoff, Landing (short final), Refueling, and Taxi (ground or air)

Flight following

- 15 min flying, 45 min sitting on the ground
- Emergency action plan activated 15 minutes after failure to report in

Example: if your aircraft took off at 1600hrs, and checked in with Air Traffic Control (ATC) at 1615hrs, the next check in time is 1630hrs. If the aircraft is 15 minutes late for check in (1645hrs) the Post Accident Emergency Action Plan is activated.

Miscellaneous CAMTS

- Required to do 5 live intubations before beginning missions
    - Quarterly intubations thereafter
- Flame retardant clothing (flight suit) – must be able to pull ¼" away from body
- Safe operation of the aircraft comes before patient care!
- Long range flights are any flight >3 hours
- The only time you don't need to wear a seat belt is during straight and level flight
    - *Or when the PIC directs you to (the PIC has ultimate authority of the mission)*

Rotary Wing Pilot in Command Qualifications

(Helicopters)

- 2,000 hours total flight time
- 1,200 hours in a helicopter
- 1,000 hours as PIC
- 100 hours as PIC at night
- MUST BE INSTRUMENT RATED (for flying IFR in IMC)
- Airline Transport Pilot (ATP) certificate is *strongly encouraged* (not required)

    - Area Orientation – 5 hours total w/ 2 at night (completed before solo mission acceptance)

Fixed Wing Pilot in Command Qualifications

(Airplanes)

- 2,000 hours total flight time
- 1,000 hours as PIC
- 100 hours at night as PIC
- Must possess an ATP certificate
- Must be instrument rated
    - Fixed wing MUST file IFR and VFR Flight Plans

FAA Rules

FAR Part 91- Applies to everyone (general FAA rules)

- No duty day
- No weather minimums (PIC assumes risk)

FAR Part 135- Flying passengers for $ (taxi services)

- Max 14 hour duty day
- 8 hours total flying time/ 8 hours "bottle to throttle" (drinking alcohol)

Weather Minimums
(CAMTS Rotorwing Standards, 05.00.000)

	Non Mountainous		Mountainous	
Condition	**Local**	**Cross Country**	**Local**	**Cross Country**
Day	800' - 2 miles	800' - 3 miles	800' - 3 miles	1000' - 3 miles
Night (w/ NVG's or TAWS)	800' - 3 miles	1000' - 3 miles	1000' - 3 miles	1000' - 5 miles

NVG's- Night Vision Goggles

TAWS- Terrain Avoidance Warning System

Marginal Weather: weather that is very close to or at minimums (can fly, but accepting risk)

Below minimums: weather that is UNDER weather minimums (can't fly)

- If bad weather is encountered while enroute, divert to the nearest facility!
- #1 cause of crashes is weather (#2 is night flight)

Flight Rules

Visual Flight Rules (VFR): This means that you can fly only in weather conditions that you can see where you are flying

- Visual Meteorological Conditions [VMC]
- There is NO intended instrument flying under these rules.

Instrument Flight Rules (IFR): This means that the weather condition do not allow safe flight by sight alone, and the pilot must be able to use his/her instruments to fly

- Instrument Meteorological Conditions [IMC]
- If the weather conditions allow VFR/VMC, a pilot may still fly under these conditions.

Inadvertent Instrument Meteorological Conditions (IIMC): This means that the pilot began flying in VFR weather and unexpectedly encountered weather that required flying by instruments.

- Referred to as *"Double IMC"*

Helicopter Landing Zones (HLZs)

Hasty or an Unsecured HLZ (Point of injury)

- Must have communication with the ground
- HLZ large enough to land (generally 100' x 100')
- *1 approach and departure heading*
- *2 Passes required prior to landing (to look for hazards on the HLZ)*
    - *One high pass, one low pass*
- If at night have two vehicles cross the beams of their headlights to mark the HLZ

Permanent Helipad (Hospital)

- Must have *2 approach and departure headings*
- Perimeter lighting on the helipad
- Landing Beacon
- Windsock

In-Flight Emergencies

- Land immediately – engine failure/fire/RPG in your tail boom
- Land as soon as possible – low transmission pressure/chip light
- Land as soon as practical – go to closest convenient place to "check something non-emergent out"

Crash Procedures

Pre-Crash Sequence

- Lay the patient flat
- Turn off any oxygen
- Assume the crash position
    - Seat belt secured
    - Sit up straight (seats are designed to absorb impact)
    - Helmet strap tight/visor down
    - Knees together, Feet 6" apart, flat on the floor
        - Not underneath the seat (they will get broken)
    - Arms crossed on chest
    - Chin to chest

Post-Crash sequence

- Turn off in order;
    - Throttle
    - Fuel
    - Battery (don't actually touch the battery though)
- Exit the aircraft (assist anyone who needs assistance)
- Assemble at the 12 o'clock position
- Begin building a shelter, build a fire, gathering water, create a signal (shelter is the first priority)
  (This is not the same as military survival priorities)

Emergency Locator Transmitter (ELT)

- Self-activates during crash sequence at 4Gs (can be manually activated)
    - Transmit frequency is 121.5 MHz
    - Upgraded transmit frequency is 406 MHz
- The ELT is what generates the constant, repeating alarm over your headset when you get near a crash site to perform a rescue

EMTALA

(Emergency **M**edical **T**reatment and **A**ctive **L**abor **A**ct)

- You must act if someone requires emergency care to sustain life or is actively giving birth
- "150 Yard rule" – if someone is injured within 150 yards of a hospital, they must be treated
- Sending physician is responsible for the patient until they arrive at next facility

Standard of Care (Negligence)

- Presence of duty
- Breach of duty
- Foreseeability
- Causation
- Injury
- Damages

Duty to Report

- Child abuse
- Elder abuse
- Violent crime

Advanced Airway Principles (5)

Intubation Indications

- Unable to swallow
- Patient can't ventilate/oxygenate
    - Failed airway algorithm
- GCS <8
- Expected clinical course
    - Inhalational burns
    - Circumferential neck or chest burns
    - Anaphylaxis
- Apnea
- Airway obstruction
    - Foreign object, maxillofacial trauma, etc.
- Respiratory failure
    - *pH <7.2, CO2 >55, PaO2 <60*
        - *only one value needs to be off to indicate the need to intubate*

LEMON

Look

Evaluate 3-3-2

- 3 fingers in mouth, 3 fingers btw jaw and hyoid, 2 fingers between hyoid and thyroid

Mallampati (I-IV)

Obstructions

Neck Mobility

Mallampati
(Airway Grading)

Mallampati I - Soft palate, uvula, anterior/posterior tonsillar pillars visible

- Tall, thin neck
- No difficulty

Mallampati II - Tonsillar Pillars hidden by tongue

- No difficulty

Mallampati III - Only the base of the uvula can be seen

- Moderate difficulty

Mallampati IV - Uvula cannot be seen

- Short, fat or muscular neck
- Severe difficulty

Intubation Review

Equipment

- Macintosh- Curved blade
    - Lifts the vallecula
- Miller- Straight blade
    - Lifts the epiglottis

Visualization Aids

Sellick's Maneuver : Direct downward pressure on the thyroid cartilage, occludes the esophagus and prevents aspiration during intubation

- DO NOT RELEASE UNTIL INTUBATION IS COMPLETE!

BURP : Backward, Upward, Rightward Pressure

- DO NOT RELEASE UNTIL INTUBATION IS COMPLETE!

Failed Airway Algorithm

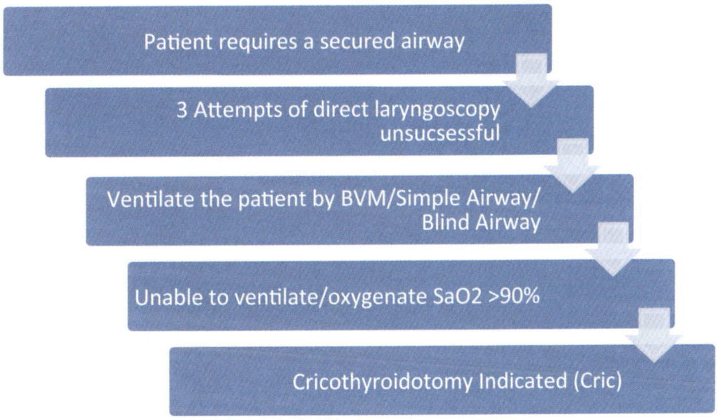

Placement Confirmation

Chest X Ray- Gold standard of placement confirmation

- Distal tip of ETT should be 2-3 cm above the carina *or;*
    - 1" above the carina
    - Level of the T2 or T3 vertebrae
- Next most reliable confirmation method- visualization of the tube passing through the vocal cords

NOTE: When inflating the distal cuff on an ETT the pressure should be between 20-30 mmHg to prevent mucosal tissue damage (only use the amount of air required to make a good seal)

Tube Check- bulb placed over the ETT after intubation to confirm placement. Remember that that esophagus is a hollow muscular tube, and will collapse around the ETT (Bulb attached to the ETT does not re-inflate if the ETT is in the esophagus)

End Tidal CO_2- if the ETT is in the trachea, there will be CO_2 in expired air (End-Tidal CO_2 or $ETCO_2$)

- Colimetric Device- a one-time use device that will change colors when CO_2 passes through it (attached to ETT)
- Capnocheck™- a reusable $ETCO_2$ device that gives both $ETCO_2$ and respiratory rate (displayed as numbers)
    - This device is now called the "EMMA Emergency Capnometer™"
    - Tip- use a finger pulse ox and an EMMA Capnometer together and you will get HR, SpO_2, RR, and $ETCO_2$
- Capnography- an electronic device attached to the ETT to measure $ETCO_2$,
    - displayed as a graph with a number value for $ETCO_2$ (see below)

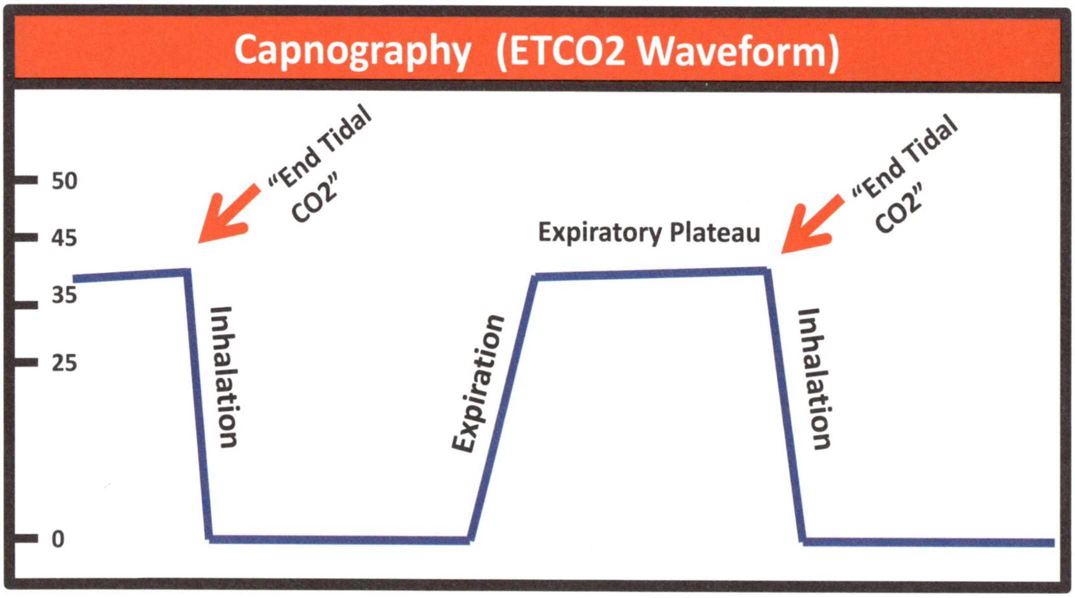

7 P's

Preparation	(Make sure equipment is serviceable)
Preoxygenate	(3-5 minutes, 10-15 LPM if possible)
Pretreatment	(LOAD, page 26)
Paralysis with induction	(Neuromuscular blockade (NMB), induction agent, and pain control)
Protect and position	(Sniffing position, place a towel under the patient's shoulder blades)
Placement with proof	(Tube passing through the vocal cords, Chest xray, Capnography, etc)
Post intubation management	(Maintain sedation, oxygenation, etc.)

LOAD

(RSI Pretreatment)

Lidocaine (Head / Lung Injury)	(blunts the cough reflex preventing ICP increase)
Opiates	(blunts the pain response)
Atropine for infants	(prevents reflexive bradycardia in infants <1 y/o)
Defasiculating Dose	(use Succinycholine, Rocuronium, or Vecuronium)

Rapid Sequence Induction/Intubation (RSI)

Neuromuscular Blockers (NMBs)

Succinylcholine (SCh) (Anectine)

- *Depolarizing* Neuromuscular Blocking (NMB)Agent
    - Causes fasiculations (muscle twitching)
    - Dose: 1 - 2 mg/kg
    - 1-2 minute onset, 4-6 minute duration
    - Can cause hyperkalemia (treat under hyperkalemia protocols)
- REQUIRES REFRIGERATION (good for 14 days once removed from refrigeration)
- Contraindications –Crush injuries, Eye injuries, Narrow angle glaucoma, History of Malignant Hyperthermia, Burns > 24 hrs., Hyperkalemia, any nervous system disorder (ex. Guillain-Barre, Myasthenia gravis)
- Can cause Malignant Hyperthermia (MH)
    - This is caused by a defect in the skeletal muscle sarcoplasmic reticulum
- Signs& Symptoms of MH:
    - Masseter spasm / trismus (lockjaw)
    - Sustained tetanic muscle contractions
    - Rapid increase in temperature (can become as high as 110^{0})
    - Increased ETCO2
    - Tachycardia / HTN
    - Mixed acidosis
- Treat with Dantrolene Sodium (Dantrium)
    - Dose 3.0 mg/kg
    - DO NOT GIVE CCBs (MH is due to a problem with Calcium removal from the cells)

Vecuronium (Norcuron)

- *Non-Depolarizing* Neuromuscular Blocking (NMB) agents
    - Does not cause fasiculations
- Used after succinylcholine to keep the patient paralyzed (slow onset, long acting)
- Defasiculating doses of a non-depolarizing agent reduces increase in ICP during intubation (LOAD)
- Slower onset (4-6 min), longer duration of action (30-45 min)
- Vecuronium Dosing:
    - 0.04-0.06 mg/kg IVP if following succinylcholine, PLUS
    - Maintenance: 0.01-0.015 mg/kg IVP 20-45min post initial PRN
- DOES NOT REQUIRE REFRIGERATION
    - It is supplied as a powder that needs reconstitution

Rocuronium (Zemeron)

- *Non-Depolarizing* Neuromuscular Blocking (NMB) agents
    - Does not cause fasiculations
- Defasiculating doses of a non-depolarizing agent reduces increase in ICP during intubation
- Used after succinylcholine to keep the patient paralyzed (slow onset, long acting)
- Slower onset (4-6 min), longer duration of action (30-45 min)
- Rocuronium Dosing
    - Maintenance: 0.1-0.2 mg/kg IV q20-30 min
- REQUIRES REFRIGERATION (good for 14 days once removed from refrigeration)
    - "Rocuronium Refrigerate"

Induction Agents
(Sedation)

Etomidate (Amidate)

Induction agent, preferred for awake sedation (because of fast onset, short half-life)

- 0.3 mg/kg
- 30-60 second onset, 3-12 minute duration

- Causes almost no change in B/P, Cardiac output, and has NO ANALGESIC PROPERTIES
    - Can have vomiting when waking up
- Contraindications- Some adrenal suppression (don't use in septic shock or Addison's Disease)

Midazolam (Versed)

- Used for Sedation/Anxiolysis with Anterograde Amnesia
    - "Helps you forget the event ever happened"
- Also useful in seizures (Versed is a Benzo)
- Dose varies based on intended use (utilize your local protocols)
    - 2.5 to 5 mg IV
    - 60-90 second onset, 15-30 minute duration
    - Use lowest dose possible, do not use with other benzodiazepine medications
- Flumazenil (Romazicon) is the reversal agent

Propofol (Diprivan)

- Hypnotic with NO ANALGESIC PROPERTIES
    - "Milk of Amnesia"
- Dose varies based on intended use (utilize your local protocols)
    - 1.5 mg/kg IV
    - 15-45 second onset, 5-10 minute duration
    - Use lowest dose possible, do not use with other benzodiazepine medications
- Decreases Cerebral Perfusion Pressure (CPP) and Mean Arterial Pressure (MAP)
    - Do not use in the patient with a head injury!
    - Not a good choice for patients that are hemodynamically unstable (in shock)
- Ketamine is a safer induction agent in shocky patients

Analgesics

Ketamine (Ketalar)

- Hypnotic (sleep producing) Analgesic (pain relieving) Amnesic (short term memory loss) drug
- Dosage varies based on intended use (utilize your local protocols)
    - 1mg/kg IV
    - 2 mg/kg IM
    - 45-60 second onset, 11-17 minute duration
- Used to stop pain impulses (remember that NMBs and Etomidate DO NOT CONTROL PAIN)
- Potent bronchodilator, use in the RSI of asthmatic patients
- Ketamine DOES NOT dry secretions in the airway (it actually can increase them)
    - If this happens (evidenced by Laryngospasm), give 0.01 mg/kg IV Atropine or 0.3mg IV Scopolamine *slowly*
- Can have hallucinations upon awakening
- Can also be given IO

Morphine

- Opiod Analgesic
- Dose based on intended use (utilize your local protocols)
    - 2 mg IV/IM/IO for mild pain control (Q4H as needed)
    - 5 mg IV/IM/IO for moderate pain control (Q4H as needed)
        - Onset within minutes, lasts 2-3 hours
    - IV is the preferred route
- Avoid in patients with head injuries and respiratory depression
    - Causes hypotension, nausea and flushing
- Often requires an antiemetic (Zofran 4mg IV/IO/IM or Phenergan 25mg IV/IO/Deep IM)
    - IV is the preferred route
- Naloxone (Narcan) 0.4-2 mg is the reversal agent (IV/IM/ via ETT)

Fentanyl

- Opiod Analgesic (100 x more powerful than morphine)
- Dose based on intended use (utilize your local protocols)
    - 50 – 100 mcg (micrograms) IV Q2H as needed
    - Also administered as a lozenge (Actiq) 400mcg or 800mcg strength
        - Actiq lozenge is only FDA approved for pain control in cancer patients (trauma use is off-label)
    - Onset within 1-2 minutes, 45-60 minute duration
- Avoid in patients with ↑ICP, hypoventilations (can cause chest wall rigidity), hypotension and bradycardia
- Often requires an antiemetic (Zofran 4mg IV/IO/IM or Phenergan 25mg IV/IO/Deep IM)
- Naloxone (Narcan) 0.4-2 mg is the reversal agent (IV/IM/ via ETT)

Ventilator Patient Management (10)

Lung Volume Definitions

Vt (Tidal Volume) = How much air the patient breathes in a normal breath

- Excessive tidal volume can cause Ventilator-Induced Lung Injury (VILI)

IRV (Inspiratory Reserve Volume) = the amount of air that can be forcefully inhaled in addition to a normal tidal volume breath

ERV (Expiratory Reserve Volume) = the amount of air that can be forcefully exhaled after a normal tidal volume breath

VC (Vital Capacity) = Tidal Volume (Vt) + Inspiratory Reserve Volume (IRV) + Expiratory Reserve Volume (ERV)

Residual Volume (RV) = the amount of air left in the respiratory tract following forceful exhalation

Total Lung Capacity (TLC) = Inspiratory Reserve Volume (IRV) + Tidal Volume (Vt) + Expiratory Reserve Volume (ERV) + Residual Volume (RV)

Dead Space= the surfaces of the airway that are not involved in gaseous exchange

- Gas exchange ONLY occurs in the alveoli
- Dead Space Formula = 2ml/kg

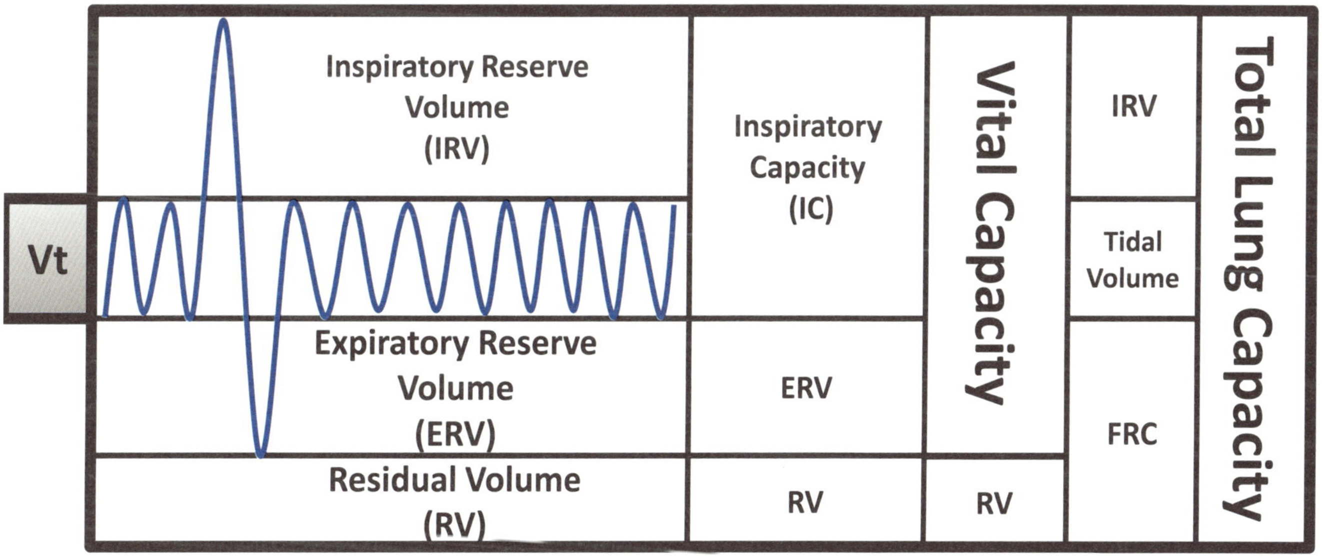

Chemoreceptors

Central- located in the medulla/pons

- Response is driven by **CO_2** and H+ levels

Peripheral- located in the aortic arch/carotid bodies

- Response is driven by **O_2**, CO2, H+
- Your bodies "pulse ox"

V/Q
(Ventilation / Perfusion)

- V/Q Scanning is a nuclear medicine study used to evaluate the circulation of air and blood within a patient's lungs in order to determine the ventilation/perfusion ratio.
    - The ventilation part of the test looks at the ability of air to reach all parts of the lungs
    - The perfusion part evaluates how well blood circulates within the lungs
    - This test is most often used to determine the presence of a pulmonary embolus (PE)

- The Fick formula is used to tell you how much O_2 a person is using
    - Formula- Cardiac output measurement based on the principle that oxygen uptake by the lungs <VO2> equals oxygen delivery

Respiratory Failure

Hypercarbic respiratory failure

"Inability to remove **CO_2**"

- Evidenced by respiratory acidosis
- Treatment- ↑ tidal volume, then the rate

Hypoxic respiratory failure

"Inability to diffuse **O_2**"

- Evidenced by low PaO_2
- Treatment - ↑ tidal volume and O_2 concentration, then the rate

Respiratory Patterns

Apneustic respirations are an abnormal pattern of breathing characterized by deep, gasping inspiration with a pause at full inspiration followed by a brief, insufficient release.

- Associated with Decerebrate Posturing

Apneustic Respirations

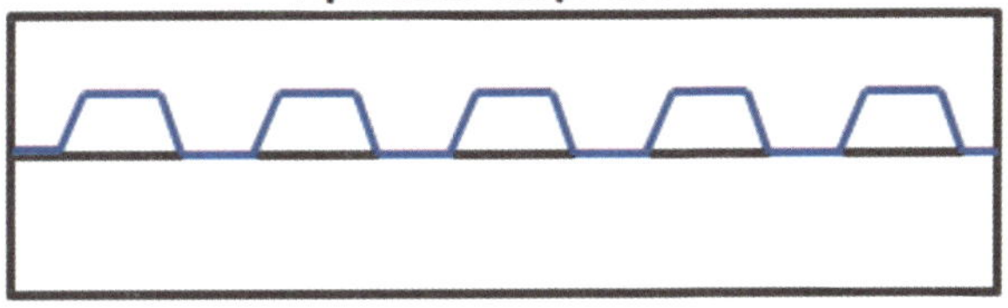

Ataxic respirations are an abnormal pattern of breathing characterized by complete irregularity of breathing, with irregular pauses and increasing periods of apnea.

- Caused by damage to the medulla secondary to trauma or stroke
- Very poor prognosis.

Ataxic Respirations

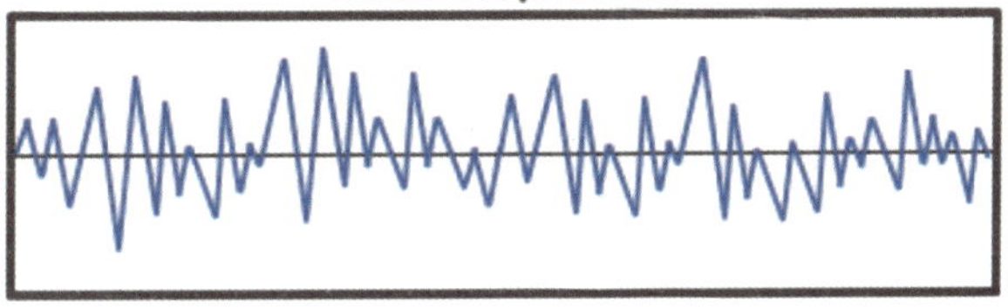

Biots respirations are an abnormal pattern of breathing characterized by groups of quick, shallow inspirations followed by regular or irregular periods of apnea

- Caused by damage to the medulla by stroke (CVA) or trauma, or pressure on the medulla secondary to brainstem herniation

Biot's Respirations

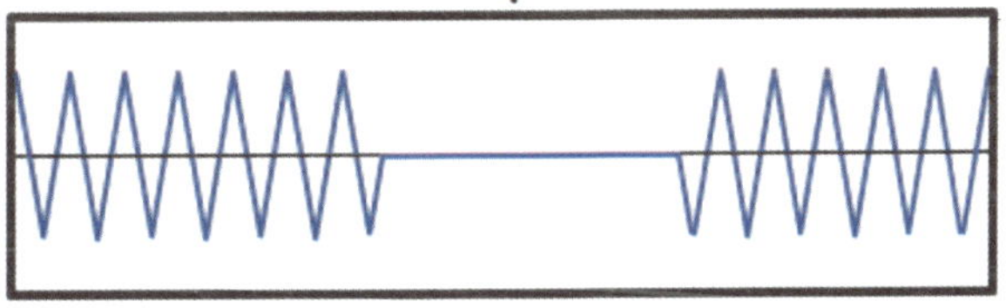

Cheyne-Stokes respirations are progressively deeper and sometimes faster breathing, followed by a gradual decrease that results in a temporary apnea

- Associated with decorticate posturing (Cushing's Δ, brainstem herniation)

Cheyne-Stoke's Respirations

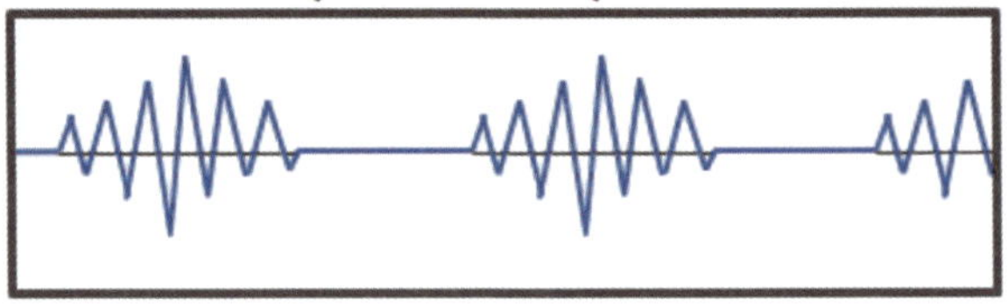

Kussmaul's respirations gradually become deep, labored and gasping

- Associated with DKA

Kussmaul's Respirations

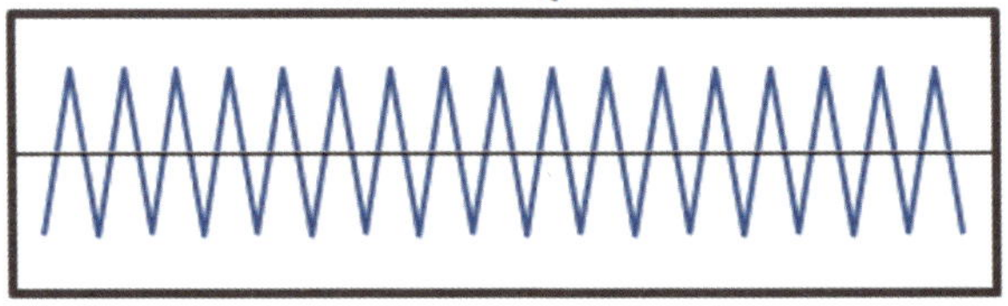

Ventilator Pearls

- The first word in the mode describes the interaction the patient has with the ventilator
    - **Controlled**- the patient's breathing rate (F) and tidal volume (Vt) is controlled completely
    - **Intermittent**- the patient can take intermittent breaths (between the controlled breaths)
    - **Synchronized**- the ventilator synchronizes delivery of breath with the patients inspiratory drive
    - **Assist**- the ventilator assists the patient with their breathing (must have intact respiratory drive)

- If on a ventilator, check tidal volume first (Vt), then the rate (F)!
    - Think of a ventilator as an automated bag valve mask (BVM). You don't start squeezing the BVM faster to increase O_2 sats; you make sure you are delivering a slow, steady squeeze to ensure quality ventilations.

- Gold Standard for **oxygenation**- pulse oximetry **(SpO_2)**
- Gold Standard for **ventilation**- capnography **($ETCO_2$)**
- Ventilator acquired pneumonia (VAP) is the #1 cause of iatrogenic death in the U.S.

Once a patient is on a ventilator, confirm settings with an ABG!

Curare Cleft Tick marks (cleft) are seen on capnography, the patient is choking, check the ETT

- Patient needs to be resedated and reparalyzed
- Use Etomidate/Versed/Propofol and Succinylcholine/Rocuronium/Vecuronium

"Curare Cleft"

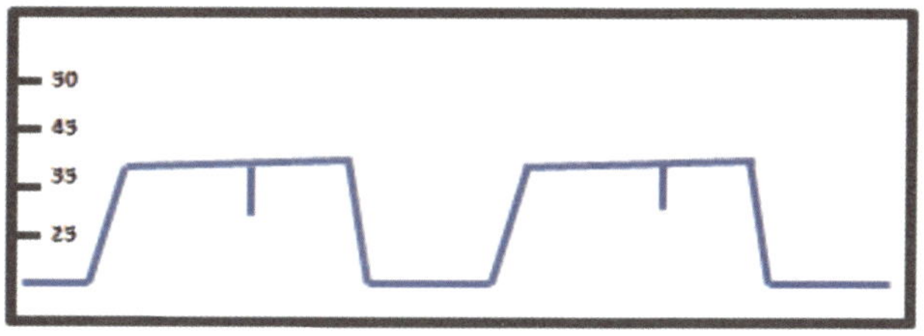

Ventilator Settings

Vt (Tidal Volume) = 6-8 cc/kg

- The volume of air delivered per breath
- Excessive Tidal Volume can lead to Ventilator-Induced Lung Injury (VILI)

F (Rate) = 8-20/min

- How many times a minute the patient is breathing (respiratory rate)

Ve (Minute Volume) = F x Vt (4-8 L/min)

- How much air is breathed by the patient in one minute

I:E (Inspiratory: Expiratory Ratio) = 1:2

- The ratio of inspiration vs. expiration (it takes longer to breath out)

FiO2 (Fraction of Inspired Oxygen) = 0.21 to 1.0 (21% - 100%)

- This ventilator feature allows for very precise delivery of oxygen concentrations
- Measuring oxygen with Liters Per Minute (LPM) is much less accurate

Pplat (Plateau Pressure) = <30

- Represents the static end inspiratory recoil pressure of the respiratory system, lung and chest wall respectively

PEEP (Positive End Expiratory Pressure) = 5

- PEEP is what keeps the alveoli open so that oxygen can diffuse
- Adequate PEEP helps prevent Atelectasis (alveolar collapse)

PEFR (Peak Expiratory Flow Rate) = **500** to 700 L/min for males, 380 to **500** L/min for females

- A person's maximum speed of expiration, as measured with a peak flow meter

Ventilator Modes

Controlled *Mandatory* Ventilation (CMV)

- Used in sedated, apneic or paralyzed patients
- All breaths are triggered, limited, and cycled by the ventilator
    - Patient has NO ability to initiate their own breaths
    - If the patient tries to take a breath in this mode they later describe it "like sucking on an empty bottle."
- Example: SAVe Ventilator

Synchronized Intermittent *Mandatory* Ventilation (SIMV)

- Assisted mechanical ventilation synchronized with the patient's breathing
    - The ventilator senses the patient taking a breath, then delivers a breath
- Spontaneous breathing by the patient occurs between the assisted mechanical breaths, which occur at preset intervals
- If the patient fails to take a breath the ventilator will provide a mechanical breath (backup rate can be set)
- This mode is preferred for patients with an intact respiratory drive
- SIMV is similar to CPAP and BPAP because they are all spontaneously triggered by the patient

Assist-Control Ventilation (AC)

- The trigger for delivery of a breath can be either the patient or elapsed time
    - Preferred mode for patients with respiratory distress
- Ventilator supports every breath, whether it's initiated by the patient or the ventilator
    - Full tidal volume (Vt) *regardless* of respiratory effort or drive
- Used in Acute respiratory distress syndrome (ARDS), paralyzed or sedated patients
- Anxious patients who frequently trigger the ventilator can hyperventilate
- *Leads to "breath stacking" or "auto-PEEP"*
    - *This can cause Ventilator-Induced Lung Injury (VILI)*

Pressure Support Ventilation (PSV)

- Pressure support makes it easier for the patient to overcome the resistance of the ET tube and is often used during weaning because it reduces the work of breathing.
    - "Supports" ventilation during inspiration
- Patient determines tidal volumes, rate (Minute Volume)
- Requires consistent ventillatory effort by the patient

CPAP/BPAP

- CPAP and BPAP are similar to SIMV because they are all spontaneously triggered by the patient

Continuous Positive Airway Pressure (CPAP) is the use of continuous positive pressure to maintain a continuous level of PEEP

- CPAP uses mild air pressure to keep an airway open

Bi-Level Continuous Positive Airway Pressure (BPAP) uses alternating levels of PEEP to maintain oxygenation, commonly used in pneumonia, COPD, asthma, etc.

- The term BiPAP™ refers to a specific manufacturer, and technically is not a ventilator mode

Pressure Alarms

Low Pressure

- Patient disconnection from machine (most common cause)
- Chest tube leaks
- Circuit leaks
- Airway leaks
- Hypovolemia

High Pressure

- Kinked line (most common cause)
- Coughing
- Secretions or mucus in the airway
- Patient biting the tube
- Reduced lung compliance (Pneumothorax, ARDS)
- Increased airway resistance

"DOPE"Ventilator Alarm Pneumonic

Dislodged	(low pressure alarm)
Obstructed	(high pressure alarm)
Pneumothorax	(high pressure alarm)
Equipment	(machine failure, dead batteries, etc.)

Preoxygenation Required]

(Give 10L/min via NRB for 15 Minutes prior to takeoff)

- Obese pt's (Bariobarotrauma)
    - Bariobarotrauma is caused by a sudden release of nitrogen stores in lipids when going to altitude
- Pregnant patients
- Pediatric patients

Personal Protective Measures

Meningitis (carried in the CSF)

- Gloves
- Mask
- Gown

Tuberculosis (carried in the sputum)

- Gloves
- Mask
- Gown
- Respirator
- Eye shield

Asthma

"The problem is breathing out"

- Decreased or absent wheezing is ominous and precedes respiratory failure
- Flattened diaphragm on Chest X-Ray (CXR), chest cavity is over expanded due to air trapping
    - *Exhalation problems fatigue the quickest!*

- Asthma exacerbation treatment
    - Increase the I:E ratio to 1:4
    - High flow O_2 (high FiO_2)
    - Bronchodilators (Albuterol, Duoneb, etc.)
    - IV Fluids

- Use Ketamine for sedation in RSI during asthma attack!
    - Ketamine is a bronchodilator

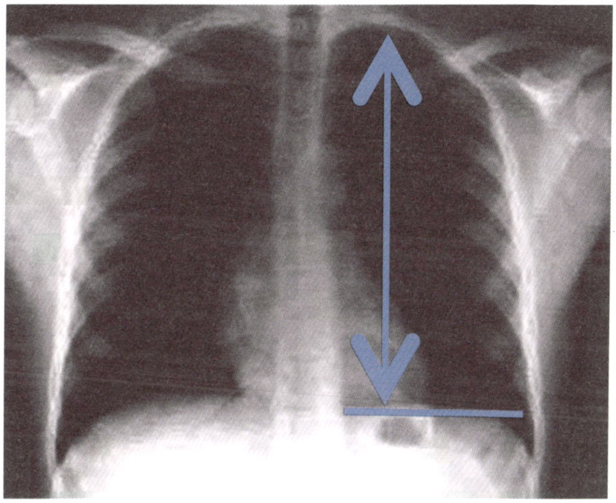

Asthma Capnogram "Shark Fin Appearance"

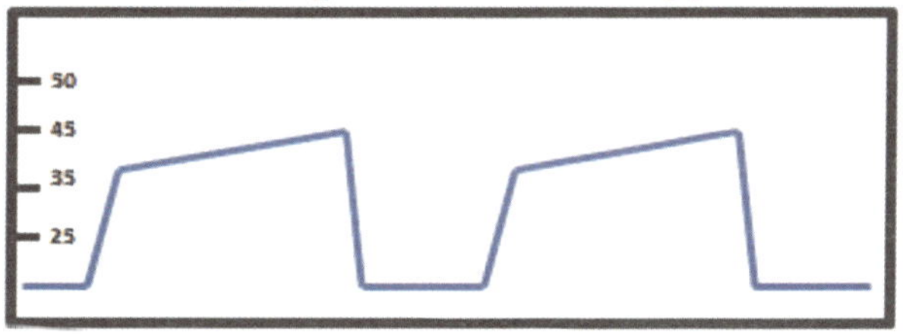

COPD

"The problem is breathing out"

- Chronic Bronchitis "blue bloaters"
- Emphysema "pink puffers"(pink color is due to polycythemia vera)

- Flattened diaphragm on CXR, chest cavity is over expanded due to air trapping
    - *Exhalation problems fatigue the quickest!*

- COPD exacerbation treatment
    - Keep FiO_2 low (hypoxic drive)
    - Nebulizer therapy (Albuterol and Ipratropium, *aka* Combivent)
    - High tidal volume (10cc/kg)
    - Increase PEEP (10)

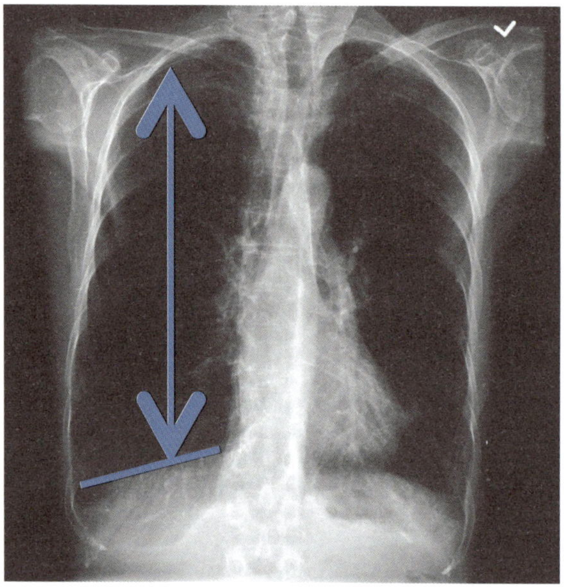

COPD Capnogram "Shark Fin Appearance"

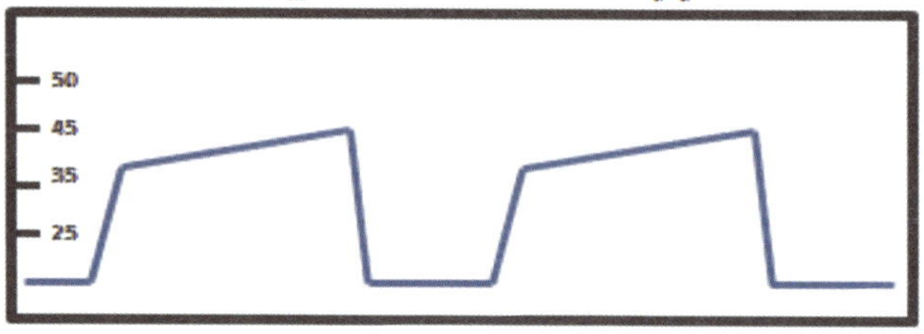

Pneumonia

- Most often viral, sometimes bacterial
- Chest X-ray (CXR) shows pleural effusions, lobar consolidation
  - Right Middle Lobe pneumonia is the most common site of consolidation
- Treat with O_2, IV Fluids, Bronchodilators, and Antibiotics if bacterial

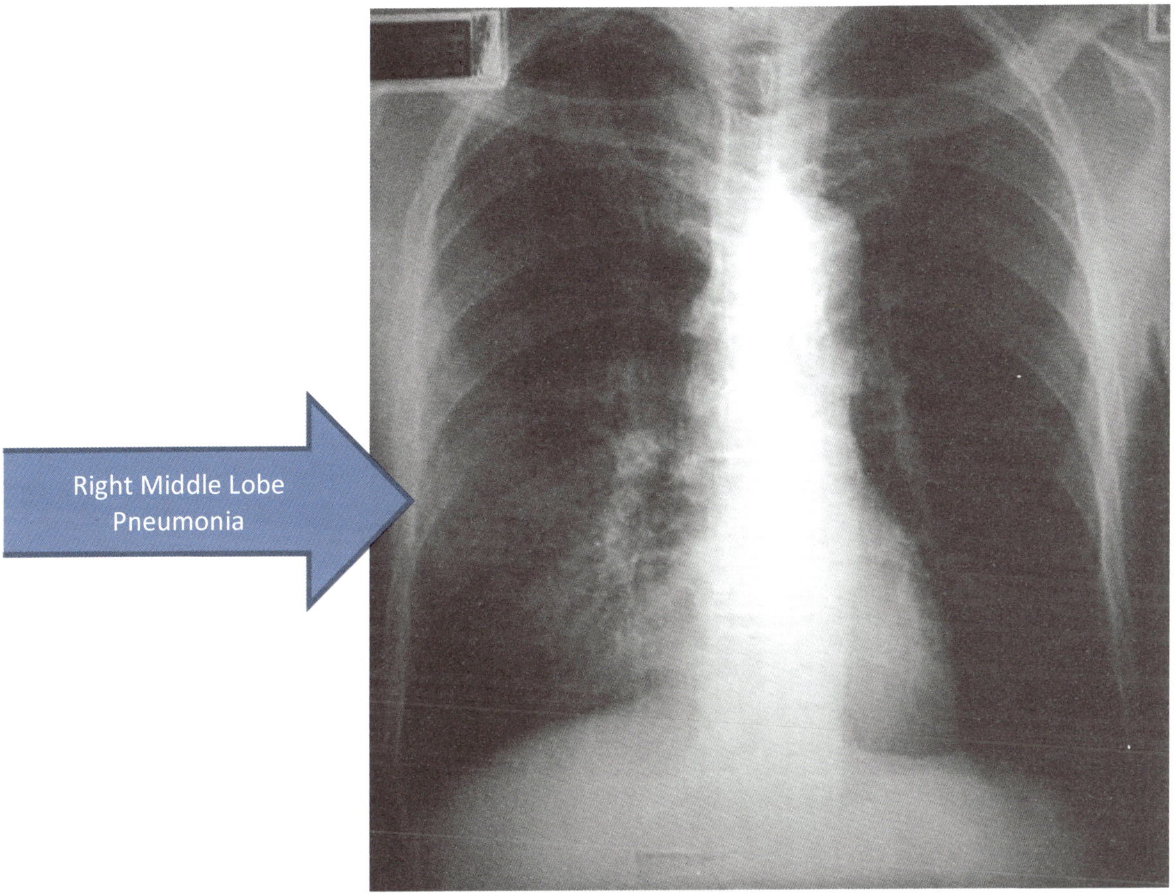

ARDS

(**A**cute **R**espiratory **D**istress **S**yndrome)

- Caused by:
  - Pancreatitis
  - Sepsis
  - Trauma
  - Aspiration Pneumonia
- Chest X-ray shows:
  - "Ground glass appearance"
  - "Patchy infiltrates"
  - "Bilateral diffuse infiltrates"
- Swann-Ganz
  - ↑PAWP (18-20)
  - This pressure is higher than normal because the Right heart is pumping against increased resistance in the lung vasculature
- Focus on oxygenation with:
  - ↑PEEP (>10)
  - High Tidal Volumes (>10cc/kg)
- Pancreatitis and ARDS commonly occur together!

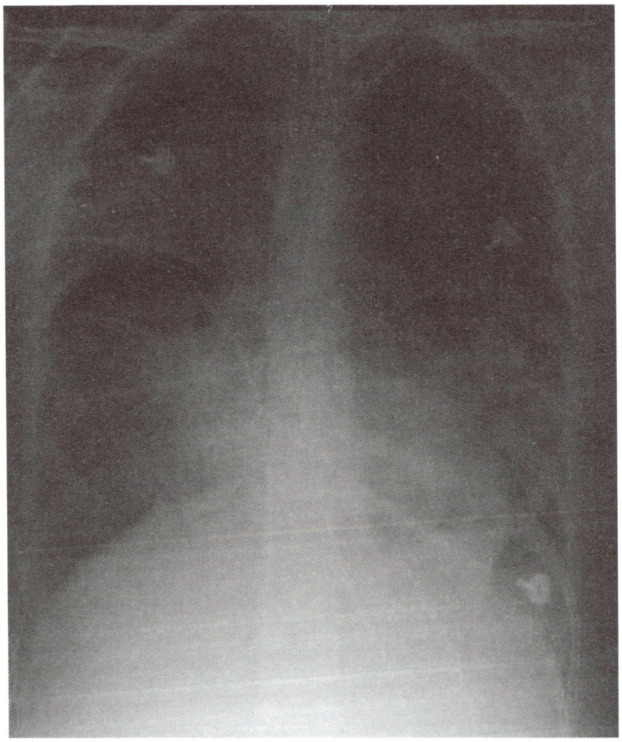

Critical Care Cardiology (20)

Cardiac Responses

In response to ↓ contractility, HR ↑

In response to hypoxia, pulmonary arteries constrict (pulmonary hypertension)

In response to a ↓ systemic perfusion, blood vessels constrict

- Except in neurogenic, spinal, septic, and anaphylactic shock!

A systemic ↑ in vasoconstriction will ↓ CO

CO (Cardiac Output) = HR x SV (4-8L/min)

By coincidence 4-8L/min is also the normal lung minute volume (Ve)

SV (Stroke Volume) is affected by preload/contractility/afterload

Preload- the load that stretches cardiac tissue BEFORE contraction

- Amount of blood returned to the right heart from the body
- Amount of blood returned to the left heart from the lungs

Contractility- the intrinsic ability of the heart/myocardium to contract

- Frank–Starling law of the heart states that the stroke volume of the heart increases in response to an increase in the volume of blood filling the heart
- The increased volume of blood stretches the ventricular wall, causing cardiac muscle to contract more forcefully

Afterload- the degree of vascular resistance to ventricular contraction

- Right heart afterload is affected by the pulmonary arteries (PVR)
- Left heart afterload is affected by systemic vascular resistance (SVR)

Cardiac Output

Pulmonary Vascular Resistance (PVR)

- Measures afterload of the Right Heart *(Normally 50-250 dynes)*
- ↑PVR: Acidosis, Hypercapnia, Hypoxia, Atelectasis, ARDS
- ↓PVR: Alkalosis, Hypocapnea, Vasodilating drugs

Systemic Vascular Resistance (SVR)

- Measures afterload of the Left Heart *(Normally 800-1200 dynes)*
- ↑SVR: Hypothermia, Hypovolemic shock, Decreased CO
- ↓SVR: Anaphylaxis , Neurogenic (distributive) shock, Septic shock, Vasodilating drugs

- ***FYI ONLY*** *- Dyne: the force required to accelerate a mass of one gram at a rate of one centimeter per second squared.*

Heart Sounds

Normal Heart Sounds

- S1 "Lub" (bicuspid/tricuspid valve closure)
- S2 "Dub" (aortic/pulmonic valve closure)

Abnormal Heart Sounds

S3 "Kentucky" Excess filling of the ventricles

- Causes: CHF, chordae tendineae (heart string) dysfunction
- CONGESTIVE HEART FAILURE IS A COMMON CAUSE!
  - S1 "Ken"
  - S2 "Tuck"
  - S3 "Y"

S4 "Tennessee" Blood being forced into a stiff (non-compliant) ventricle

- Causes: Hypertrophic cardiomyopathy, Hypertension (HTN)
- ASSOCIATED WITH MYOCARDIAL INFARCTION!
  - S4 "Tenn"
  - S1 "E"
  - S2 "See"

Auscultation Points

- Aortic
- Pulmonic
- Tricuspid
- Mitral
  - Murmur Grading: Grade I – Barely Audible, Grade VI– Loud

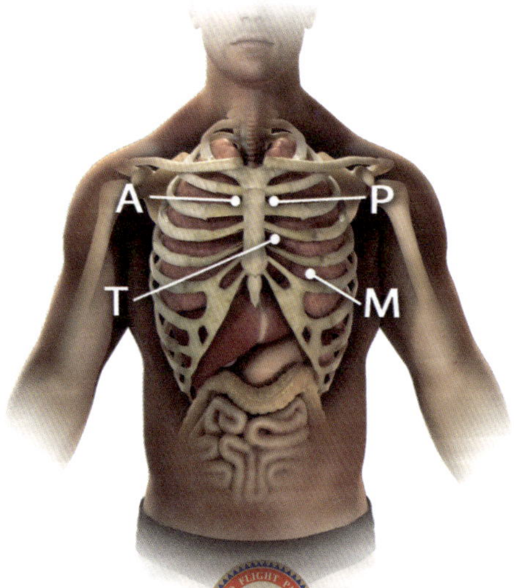

Coronary Circulation

Right Coronary Artery (RCA)

RCA

- Supplies the right ventricle and in most of the population the SA Node (60%)
- Inferior MI
- Bradycardia due to SA node involvement

Posterior Descending Artery (PDA)

- A branch off of the RCA in most of the population (85%)
- Inferior wall
- Ventricular septum
- Papillary muscles ("heart-strings")

Left Coronary Artery (LCA)

- A complete block of the LCA is called the "widow maker" because it occludes both the LAD and LCX (basically the entire left heart). Sometimes referred to as the "Left Main Artery"

Left Anterior Descending (LAD)

- Supplies anterior left ventricle/ anterior septum
- Anterior MI/ Septal MI/ Anterospetal MI

Left Circumflex (LCX)

- Sometimes called the "Circumflex Artery"
- Supplies lateral Left ventricle/ posterior left vent in 45% of population
- Lateral MI/ Posterior MI

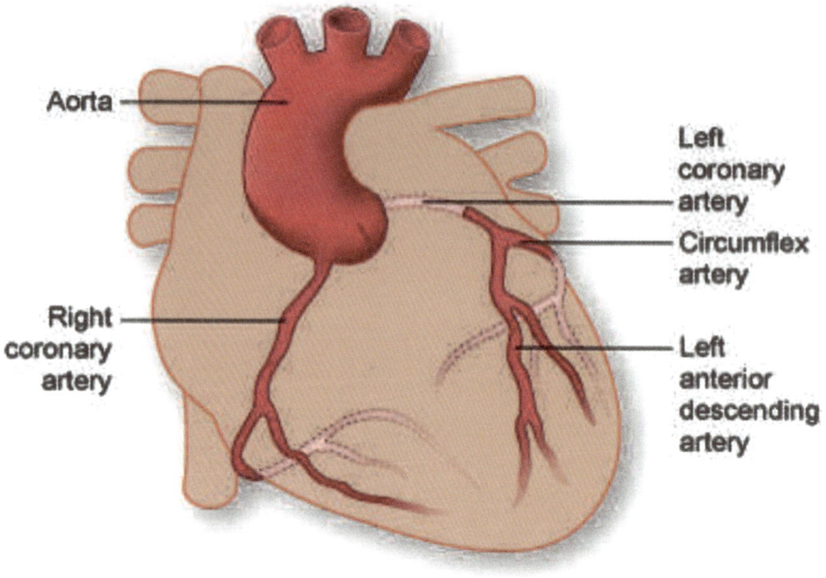

Acute Coronary Syndromes

STEMI (ST Segment Elevation Myocardial Infarction)

- ST Elevation in 2 contiguous leads >2mm
- "Cardiac death happening now"
    - "Time is muscle"
- Often associated with new onset LBBB – (widened QRS, downward deflection in V1)
- (+) Positive cardiac markers/enzymes

Non-STEMI

- ST Depression or dynamic T wave changes in 2 contiguous leads
    - ST Depression is caused by a lack of O2 to cardiac tissue (either occurring now or due to an old infarct)
    - Dynamic T wave changes are T wave inversion (point down instead of up)
- (+) Positive Cardiac markers/enzymes

Unstable Angina

- Angina that **is not** relieved by rest, nitro, or is different quality that the patients "normal" chest pain
- May have ST segment depression

Progression of EKG Changes in Myocardial Infarction

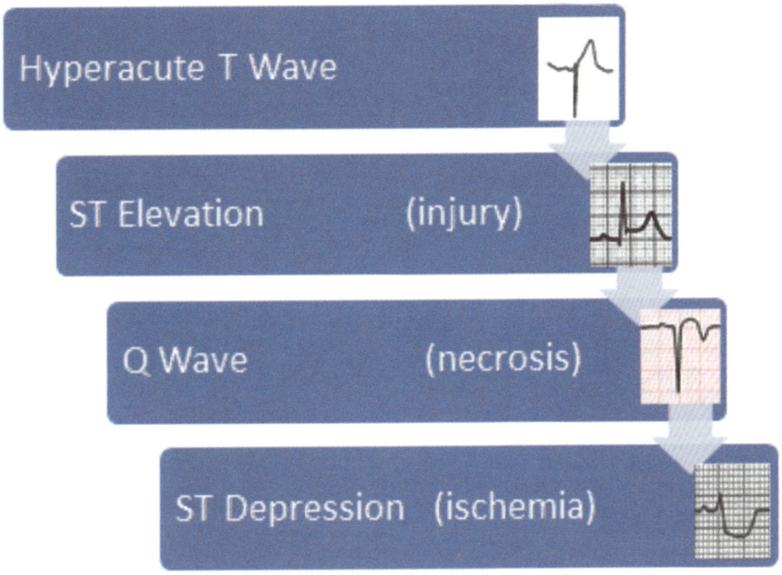

Cardiac Enzymes

Cardiac Panel= Troponin I, CK-MB, MB

- This panel is run at set intervals (content and time based on local facility protocols)

Enzyme/Marker	Specificity	Detectable at	Peak Levels
Troponin I	High	2 hours	12 hours
Creatinine Kinase Myoglobin (CK-MB)	Moderate	4 to 8 hours	12 to 24 hours
Myoglobin (MB)	Low	3 hours	4 to 9 hours

How to approach the 12 lead EKG

- Be consistent in your approach! The 12 lead EKG can be daunting, but remember that you are a good Paramedic. As a Paramedic, you are used to seeing rhythm strips in lead II. Identify the things you know to be normal/abnormal, then look at 12 lead EKG for ST Segment appearance (normal, elevated, depressed).

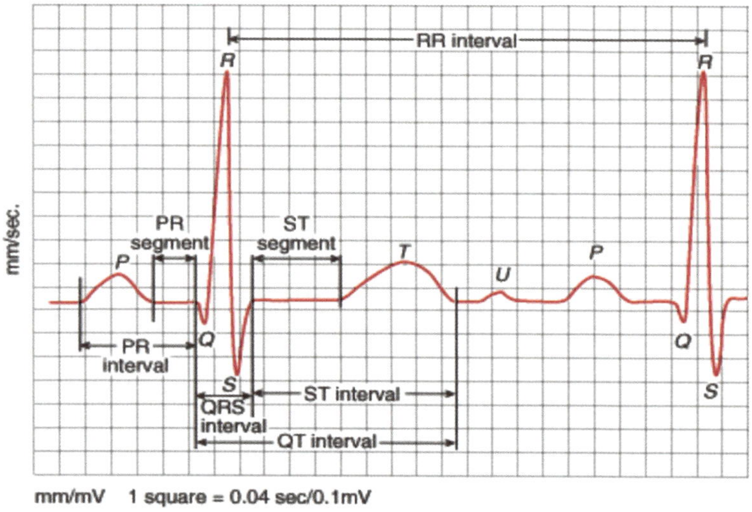

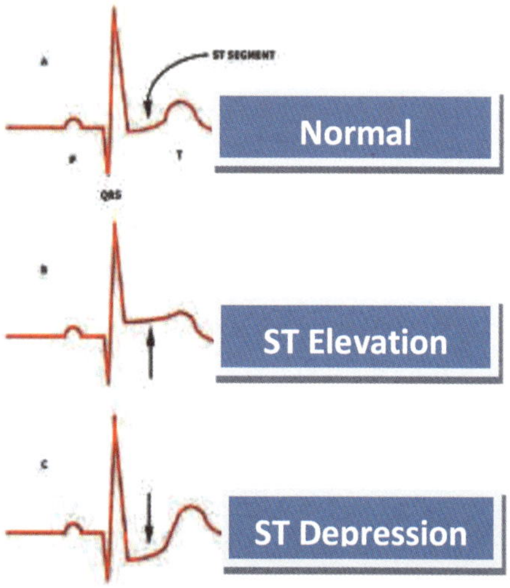

- Think of the EKG as a camera. The heart doesn't change its location, the angle of the camera changes (example: lead I, II, III, V_1, V_2, etc.)

- Always follow the same pattern. I look for Inferior, Anteroseptal, and then a Lateral MI. If you don't see anything there, dig deeper with the "PAILS" approach (chart below).
    1. II, III, aVF (Inferior MI)
    2. V_1, V_2, V_3, V_4 (Anteroseptal MI)
    3. I, aVL, V_5, V_6 (Lateral MI)

Location	EKG Leads	Vessel Affected	Treatment
Posterior	Reciprocal Changes V_1, V_2, V_3, V_4	LCX	MONA
Anterior	V_2, V_3, V_4	LAD	MONA
Inferior	II, III, aVF	RCA	2L Fluid Challenge NO Nitro or Beta Blockers
Lateral	I, aVL, V_5, V_6	LCX	MONA
Septal	V_1, V_2	LAD	MONA

Posterior MI
(LCX)

- Reciprocal EKG changes in V1, V2, V3, V4
    - Reciprocal change = Inverted QRS Complex or ST segment depression
- ST depression predominantly in V1, V2
- Treat with MONA

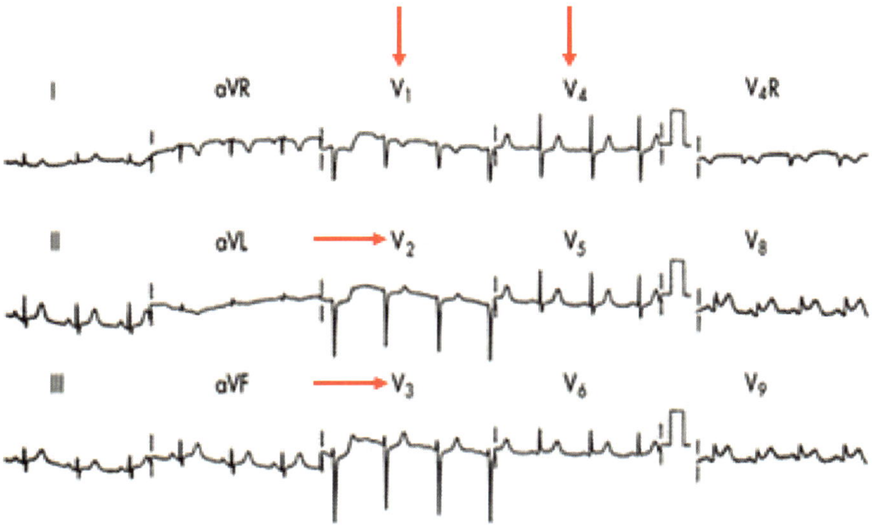

Anterior MI
(LAD)

- ST segment changes in V2, V3, V4
- Treat with MONA

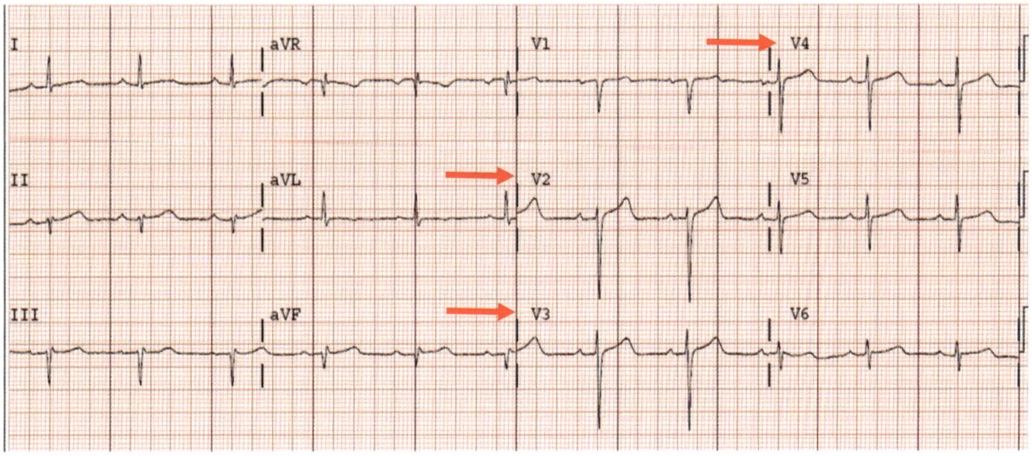

Inferior MI
(RCA)

- ST segment changes in II, III, aVF
- Papillary muscle "heart strings" dysfunction
- GET A RIGHT SIDED EKG! (RV4)
- Can cause Bradycardia, 1°,2° AV Block
- Treatment - 2L fluid challenge
    - No nitro or Beta blockers!

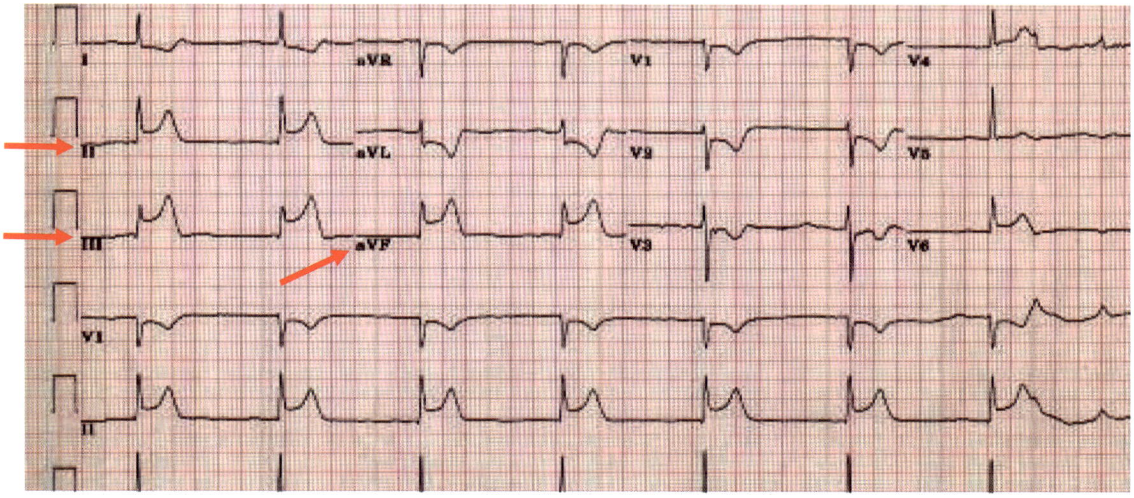

Lateral MI
(LCX)

- Lateral/Posterior Wall ST segment changes in 1, V5, V6, aVL
- Treat with MONA

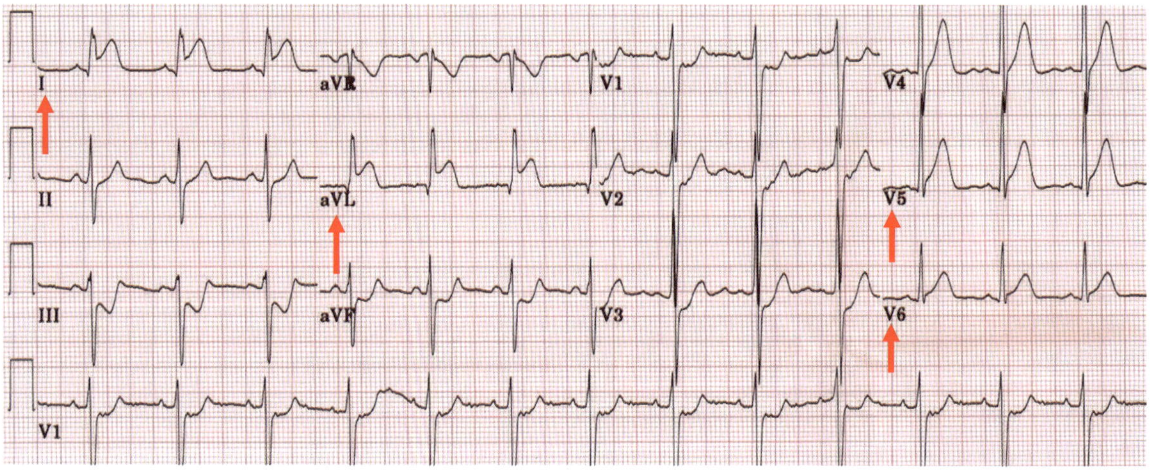

Anteroseptal MI
(LAD)

- ST segment changes in V1,V2,V3,V4
- Left ventricle and septum affected
- Papillary muscle dysfunction- leads to cardiogenic shock
- Treat with MONA

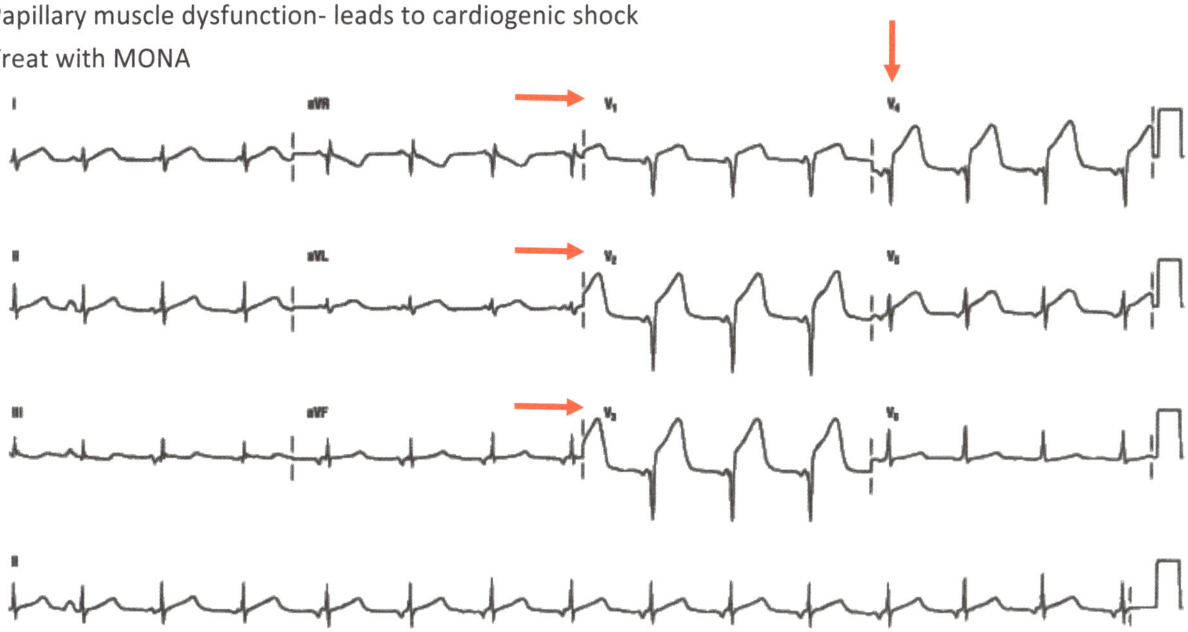

Summary of EKG Changes

This can be placed directly over a 12 lead EKG to correlate area of infarct

I Lateral	aVR	V1 Septal	V4 Anterior
II Inferior	aVL Lateral	V2 Septal	V5 Lateral
III Inferior	aVF Inferior	V3 Anterior	V6 Lateral

Summary of Vessels & Treatment

LCX MONA	aVR	LAD MONA	LAD MONA
RCA 2L Fluids	LCX MONA	LAD MONA	LCX MONA
RCA 2L Fluids	RCA 2L Fluids	LAD MONA	LCX MONA

Bundle Branch Blocks

- Caused by a defect in electrical impulse conduction (slows conduction)
  - Widened QRS (>0.12 sec), or "Rabbit Ears
- Look at V1 for changes
  - Think of the turn signal in your car. To make a right turn you flip the turn signal up (Right Bundle Branch Block). To make a left turn you flip the turn signal down (Left Bundle Branch Block)

Right BBB Amplitude **UP**

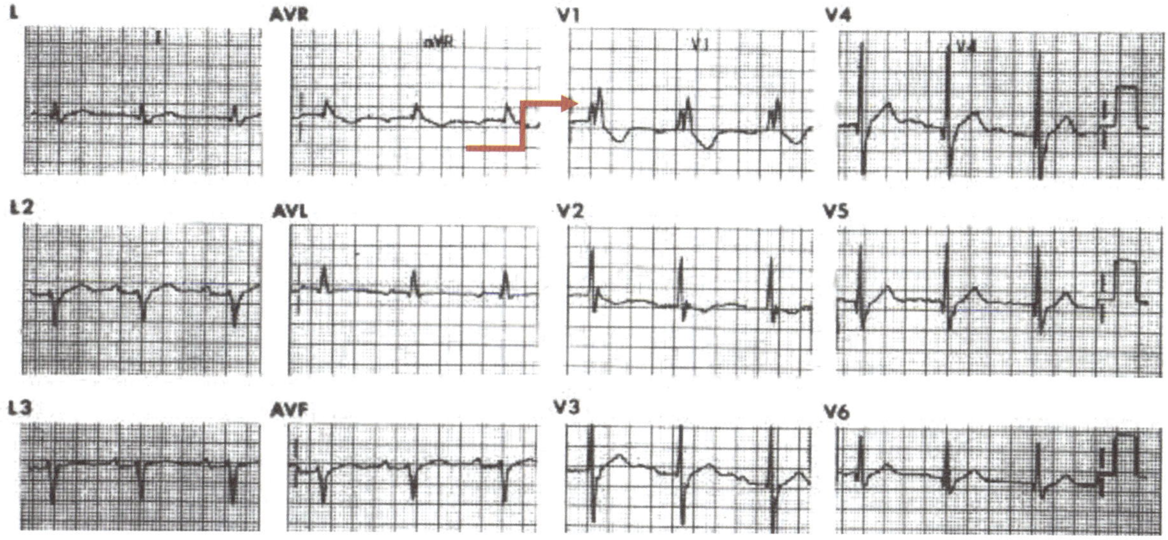

Left BBB Amplitude **DOWN**

Associated with new onset AMI

Look for elevated cardiac enzymes

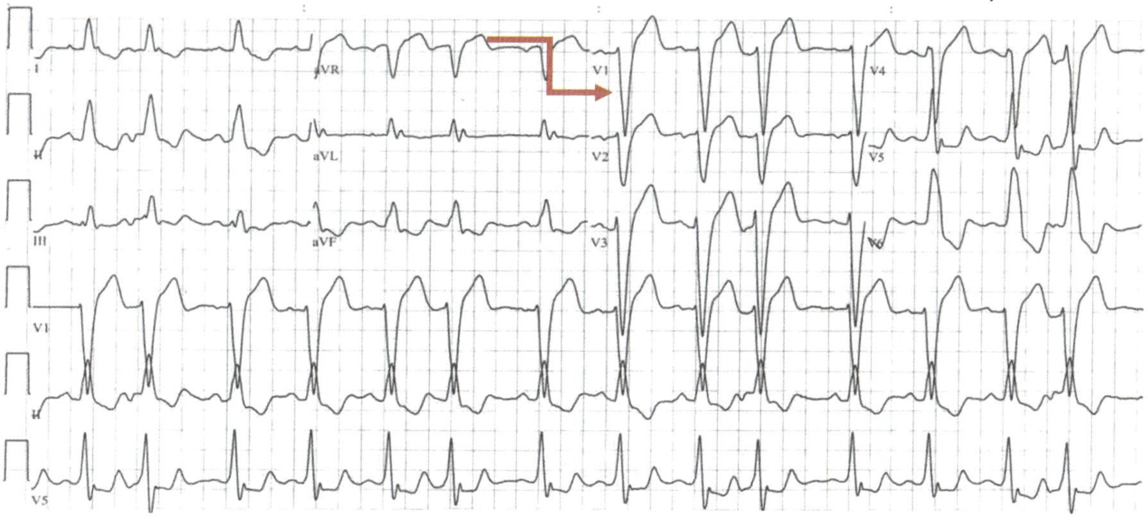

AMI Treatment

- Reduce Preload/Pain ("MONA")
- Reduce HR/O2 demand (Beta Blockers/CCBs)
- Clot Prevention (ASA)
- Reperfusion (Chemical or Surgical)

"MONA"

- Morphine, Oxygen, Nitro, ASA (Aspirin)

Beta Blockers

- Reduces heart rate, thus reduces myocardial oxygen demand
- DO NOT use in bi-fasicular blocks or BBB

Heparin/Low Molecular Weight Heparin (Lovenox)

- Prevents fibrinogen conversion to fibrin to decrease clot formation in the coronary arteries

Angiotensin Converting Enzyme Inhibitors (ACEi)

- Prevents ventricular remodeling in the Post-MI patient (keeps heart muscle from growing too much to make up for lost tissue from MI

ACLS Drug Chart

Drug	Indication	Dosage
Adenosine	Narrow Complex SVT	6mg / 12mg / 12mg
Amiodarone	V/F & Pulseless V tach	300mg 1st dose / 150mg 2nd dose
Atropine	Sinus Bradycardia &Organophosphate Poisoning	0.5mg q3min (max 3mg)
Dopamine	2nd Line for Bradycardia & Hypotension (<70 SBP)	2-20mcg / kg / min
Defibrillation	V/F & Pulseless V tach	120J then 200J Biphasic or 200J then 360J Monophasic
Epinephrine	VF / Pulseless VT / Asystole / PEA	1mg (1:10,000) q3-5min
Lidocaine	Alternative to Amiodarone	1.0 - 1.5 mg / kg (max 3mg / kg)
Magnesium Sulfate	Torsades De Pointe & Arrhythmia 2° to Digitalis	1 - 2 grams (over 30 - 60 min)
Vasopressin	Alternative pressor to Epi / Septic Shock	40 units x 1 dose

Narcan, Atropine, Epinephrine, Lidocaine and Vasopressin can be given via ETT (increase the dose 2 – 2.5 x normal)
Defibrillation in-flight is safe, be sure to use standard precautions and inform the pilot

Antidysrythmics

Class I (Sodium Channel Blockers)

- Lidocaine, Phenytoin, Procainamide
- Interferes with Sodium (Na+) channels

Class II (Beta Blockers)

- Carvedilol, Labetolol, Propanolol, Timolol, Esmolol, Metoprolol
- Anti-sympathetic nervous system agents
- Beta Blockers- reduce heart rate, reduce cardiac oxygen demand
    - Do not use if patient has a heart block or Inferior MI (II, III, aVF)

Class III (Miscellaneous)

- Amiodarone
- Affects potassium (K+) efflux

Class IV (Calcium Channel Blockers)

- Verapamil, Diltiazem, Cardizem
- Affects the AV Node

Class V (Other)

- Adenosine, Digoxin, Magnesium Sulfate
- Works by "other" mechanisms (no good way to classify/stratify the meds)

Neurovascular System Refresher

- α1- Vasoconstrict
- β1- increase heart rate, contractility
- β2- Dilate bronchioles/ blood vessels
- Dopaminergic – gut kidney vessel dilation
- Cholinergic – decrease heart rate

Pneumonic: You have one heart and two lungs (β_1 affects the heart, β_2 affects the Lungs)

Vasoactive Drugs

↑ SVR (Systemic Vascular Resistance): Dopamine, Neo-synephrine, Epinephrine, Levophed

- NorEpi (Levophed) - used for patients in profound hypotension

↓ SVR (Systemic Vascular Resistance): Nitroprusside (Nipride), High Dose NTG, CCBs, ACEi, α Blockers, Dobutrex, Natrecor

- Nitroprusside (Nipride) - reduces preload and afterload by dilation (can cause cyanide toxicity)
  - *THIS IS NOT THE SAME AS NITROGLYCERIN!*
- Nicardipine – reduces afterload (does not cause cyanide toxicity)

↑ Preload: Vasoconstrictors (drugs that ↑SVR), fluids

↓ Preload: Vasodilators, Morphine, Lasix, Nitro (drugs that ↓ SVR)

↑ SVR *Vasoconstrictors*	**↓ SVR** *Vasodilators*	**↑ Preload** *Vasoconstrictors*	**↓ Preload** *Vasodilators*
Dopamine Neo-synephrine Epinephrine **Levophed**	**Nitroprusside (Nipride)** Nicardipine High Dose Nitro CCBs Natrecor	Dopamine Neo-synephrine Epinephrine **Levophed** **Fluids**	**Morphine** **Lasix** **Nitro**

Diuretics and Vasodilators make cardiac output worse (Lasix, Morphine, Nitro)

Fibrinolytics

(Chemical reperfusion breaks the clot)

Indications

- Clinical presentation consistent with AMI within **12hrs** of Sx onset
- EKG showing ST elevation (STEMI) in ≥2 leads or new onset LBBB
- Absence of contraindications
- Absence of cardiogenic shock

Absolute Contraindications (think of the contraindications like a non-compressible hemorrhage)

- Prior intracranial hemorrhage (ICH)
- Known structural cerebral vascular lesion
- Known malignant intracranial neoplasm
- Ischemic stroke within 3 months
- Suspected aortic dissection
- Active bleeding or bleeding diathesis (excluding menses)
- Significant closed-head trauma or facial trauma within 3 months

Relative Contraindications

- History of chronic, severe, poorly controlled hypertension
- Severe uncontrolled hypertension on presentation (SBP >180 mm Hg or DBP >110 mm Hg)
- Traumatic or prolonged (>10 min) CPR or major surgery less than 3 weeks
- Recent (within 2-4 week) internal bleeding
- Non-compressible vascular punctures
- For streptokinase/anistreplase - Prior exposure (more than 5 days ago) or prior allergic reaction to these agents
- Pregnancy
- Active peptic ulcer
- Current use of anticoagulant (Warfarin, Heparin, Lovenox, etc.)

Surgical Reperfusion

PTCA

Percutaneous Trans luminal Coronary Angioplasty "Cardiac Cath"

- Administer GP2B3A inhibitors
    - This class of medications prevents platelet activity. The difference between this medication and Aspirin (Thromboxane A2 inhibitor) is that aspirin irreversibly binds for 3-5 days, whereas GP2B3A inhibitors can be titrated and have a half-life of about 8 hours (binding stops when half-life ends).
    - GP2B3A examples- Reopro, Integrilin, Aggrastat

- Keep the leg straight during transport and hold direct pressure for 30 minutes after cardiac catheter removal
    - This is to prevent the femoral artery from re-bleeding

CABG

Coronary Artery Bypass Graft "Cardiac Bypass"

- RCA (Right Coronary Artery)-repaired using the Saphenous Vein
- LAD (Left Anterior Descending)- repaired using the Inferior Mammary Artery (IMA)
    - Used for multiple vessel disease, Left Coronary Artery (LCA) disease
    - The LCA is sometimes referred to as the "Left Main" or "Widomaker"

"Other" Coronary Problems

Angina

Stable- Discomfort /Pain lasting 1 to 5 minutes, relieved by rest, nitro, *predictable course*

Variant (Prinzmetals)

- Chest pain at rest, has a circadian rhythm (most often in the early morning)
- Most often seen in women
- Treated with Nitro and Calcium channel blockers (CCBs)

Silent- no pain, but objective evidence of ischemia on EKG (ST depression)

Heart Transplant

- If a heart transplant patient is decompensating, immediate cardioversion is indicated
- Dopamine and Normal Saline fluid bolus should be used in the setting of bradycardia
    - Can also use Neosynephrine (sympathomimetic)
    - DO NOT use atropine (it won't work)

Wolff-Parkinson-White Syndrome (WPW)

- Heart condition in which there is an extra electrical circuit in the heart (causes tachycardia)
- One of the most common causes of fast heart rate disorders in infants and children
- Treated by surgical ablation of the errant pathway (see yellow arrows)
- Causes a "delta wave" on EKG (see red arrow)

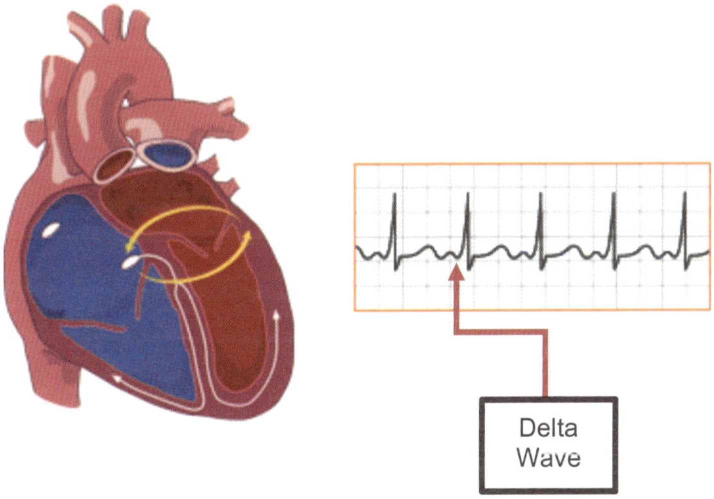

Endocarditis

- Inflammation or infection on the inside of the heart (endo = inside)
- Sudden onset infection with *NEW MURMUR*
- #1 cause is IV Drug abuse
- Osler Nodes (painful red fingertips)
- Janeway Lesions (red lesions on the palm and soles)

Often treated with IV antibiotics and sometimes heart valve replacement if damage is severe enough

Pericarditis

- Inflammation or infection on the outside of the heart (peri = around)
- Substernal chest pain when breathing or laying supine (pericardium rubs against the sternum)
    - Most common cause is Idiopathic (80%)
        - Idiopathic means the cause can't be identified

Uremic Pericarditis: Can be seen in the patient that is undergoing dialysis because they are in renal failure
Dressler's Syndrome: Pericarditis occurring in the post MI/ post cardiac surgery patient

- Global ST Elevation(see EKG below), rounded T waves
    - *Also known as diffuse ST Segment elevation*
- Treated with NSAIDS (usually Indocin)
    - Colchicine is rapidly becoming the treatment of choice for pericarditis (gout medication)

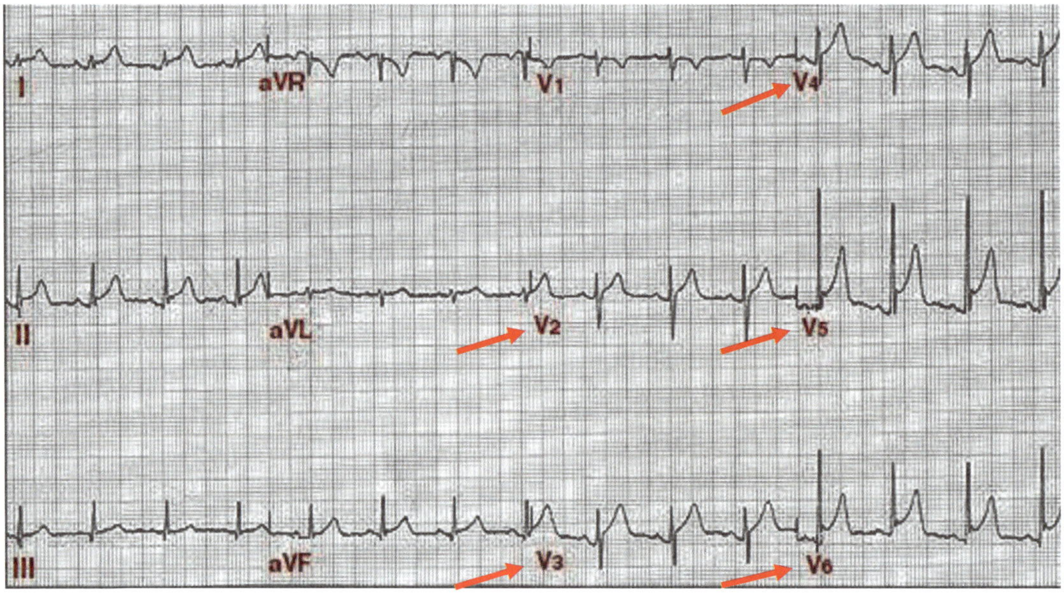

Congestive Heart Failure (CHF)

- Patient presents with progressive dyspnea, coughing up frothy sputum, etc.
    - Most common cause of right heart failure is left heart failure
- Butterfly pattern/ Kerley B Lines, Bilateral Diffuse Infiltrates
- Heart >50% width of chest (heart width is between blue lines below)

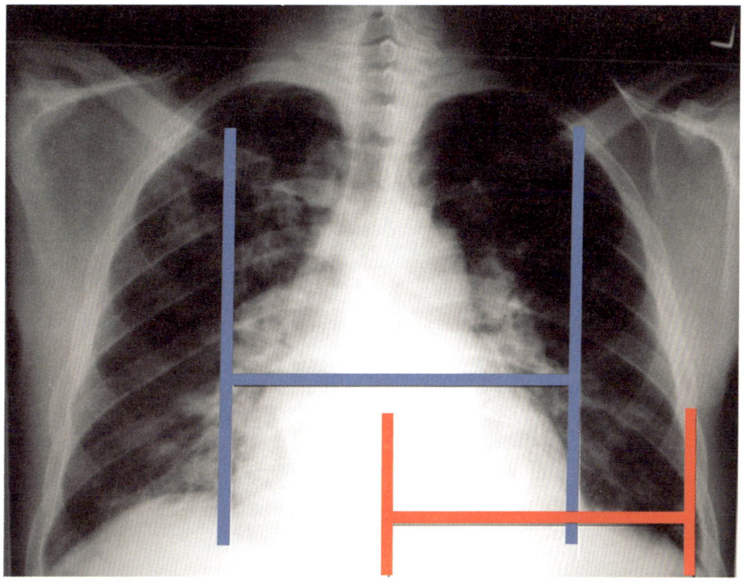

- BNP (B-type Natriuretic Peptide) increase on blood work. BNP is released by the ventricles in response to stretching and causes diuresis, reducing preload and afterload
    - *Natrecor* (Nesiritide) *is synthetic BNP*

BNP Level	Clinical Correlation
< 100 pg/mL	No Heart Failure
>300 pg/mL	Mild Heart Failure
>600 pg/mL	Moderate Heart Failure
>900 pg/Ml	Severe Heart Failure

Pg/mL- picograms per milliliter

Treatment

- **Lasix is the most important drug therapy (high dose)**
- Nitroglycerin (second most important drug therapy)
- CPAP/BPAP is often used to decrease work of breathing (WOB)
- ACEi (Angiotensin Converting Enzyme inhibitor) to prevent ventricular remodeling (Enalipril, Captopril)
- Beta blockers (Carvidolol)

Aortic Dissection

- Described as a "Ripping or Tearing" sensation between the shoulder blades
  - Pain can also present in the chest or abdomen, still described as "ripping or tearing"
  - Common with Marfan's syndrome
  - Ascending Aorta most common site of dissection
  - CXR shows widened mediastinum, loss of aortic knob, pleural effusion

- A difference of 20 mmHg Systolic B/P in the arms is a common finding with dissection

- Treat FIRST with β Blockers (**Labetalol [Normodyne]**), then Vasodilators (**Nitroprusside [Nipride])**
  - DO NOT USE NITROPRUSSIDE *FIRST* BECAUSE IT CAUSES REFLEX TACHYCARDIA!
- Pain meds
  - Morphine, Fentanyl, Ketamine
- Restrict fluids unless hypotensive

Aortic Aneurysm

- NOT THE SAME AS DISSECTION!
  - Aneurysm is an "out pouching" of either the cardiac aorta or the abdominal aorta
- Typically found on routine CT scans for other medical problems or during physical exam (abdominal aorta palpation >5cm).
  - Surgically repaired when >5cm, or symptomatic

Hemodynamic Monitoring

(Monitored with a Swann Ganz Catheter)

A Swan-Ganz catheter is used to measure how much pressure blood is under when it goes into the pulmonary artery. It also provides measurements of right heart afterload and left heart preload. A pulmonary artery catheter and Swann-Ganz Catheter utilize the same vascular access site (central line in the subclavian vein).

- Distal tip is used to measure pressures
- Do not exceed 1.5cc air in distal cuff
- Do not take wedge pressure readings for >15 seconds or 3 breaths
- Take readings at the end of exhalation
- PA port only for monitoring /lab sample blood draw (not fluid resuscitation)
- When transporting a patient with a PA catheter, deflate the balloon(prevents an inadvertent wedge pressure)
    - This is because the balloon size increases at altitude due to Boyle's Law

Note: There are several terms that describe the pressure readings in regards to the Swan Ganz. The terms below are describing the same reading!

PAWP (Pulmonary Artery Wedge Pressure)
PAOP (Pulmonary Artery Occlusion Pressure)
PACP (Pulmonary Artery Capillary Pressure)

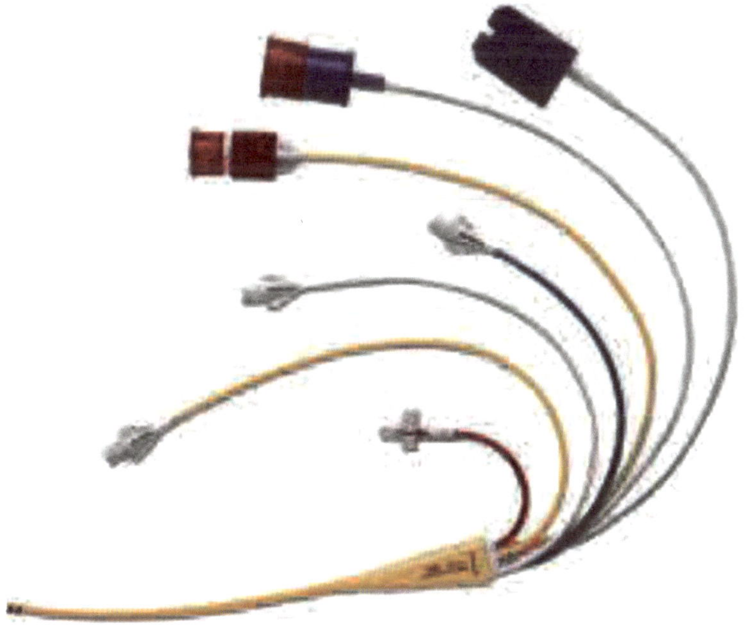

Swan Ganz Progression

1. Passing through the Right Atrium (from the subclavian)
2. Passing into the Right Ventricle
3. Final destination, the Pulmonary Artery
4. Balloon inflated to get a "Pulmonary Artery Wedge Pressure" (PAWP)

    Remember- PAWP, PCWP, and PAOP are the SAME THING

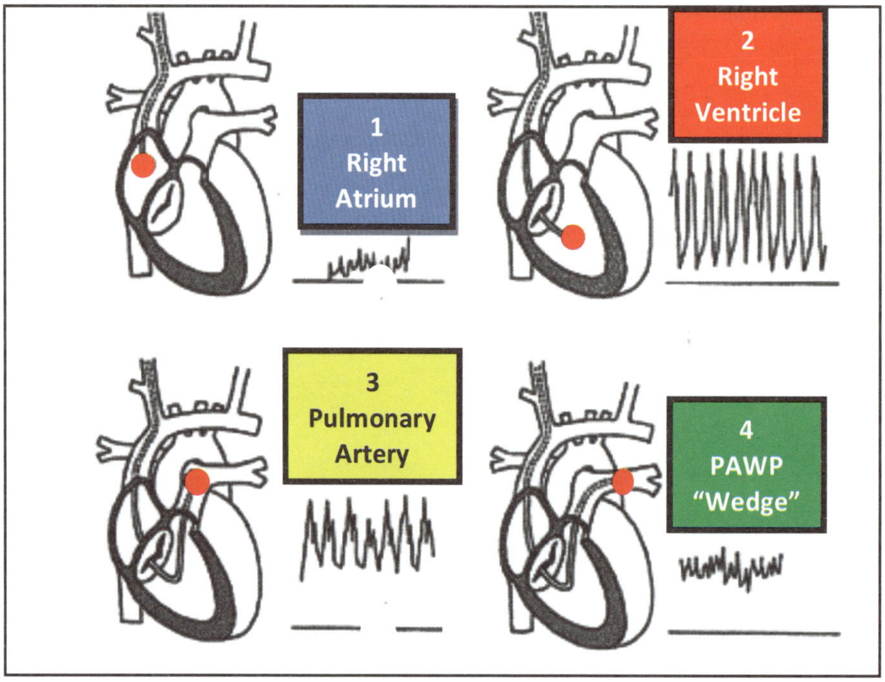

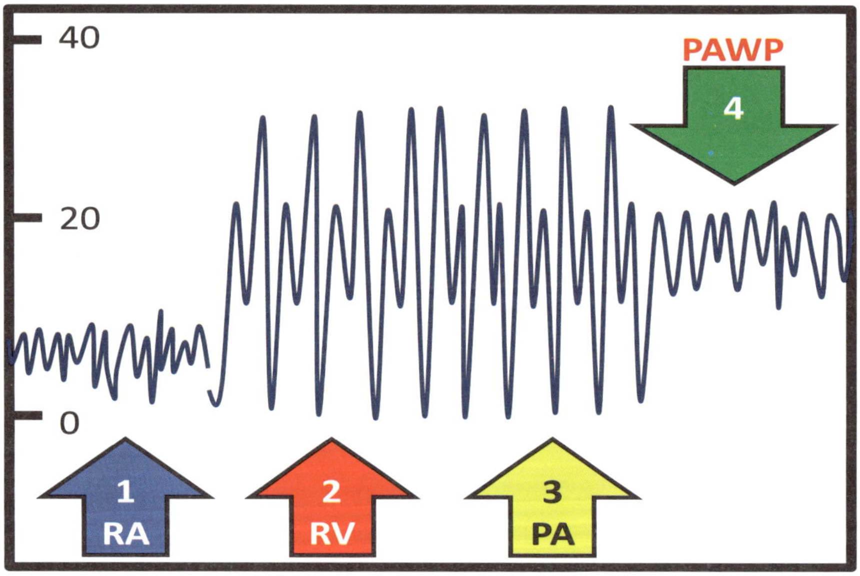

Normal Values

CVP (Central Venous Pressure)

"Right Atrial Pressure"

- Measures Right heart preload
    - Normal = 2 to 6 mmHg

RV (Right Ventricular pressure)

- Right Heart Afterload
    - 15-25mmHg systolic
    - 0-5 mmHg diastolic

PA (Pulmonary Artery pressure)

- 15-25mmHg systolic
- 8-15 mmHg diastolic

PAWP (Pulmonary Artery Wedge Pressure)

Wedge Pressure

- Measures Right heart afterload
- Measures Left heart preload
    - 8-12 mmHg

CO (Cardiac Output)

- 4-6 L/min

Coronary Perfusion Pressure (CPP)

- DBP-PCWP
    - 50-60 mmHg

Right Ventricular Waveform

Right Ventricular Pressure **(RV)**

- 15-25mmHg systolic
- 0-5 mmHg diastolic
- This waveform may or may not have a Dicrotic notch on the left
  - Referred to as a "high amplitude waveform"

Catheter Whip- If the monitor shows this waveform, the tip of the catheter needs to be "floated" into the PA. Allowing the catheter to remain in the right ventricle may result in V-Fib

- Inflate the cuff with 1.5 cc of air
- Have the patient cough
- Lay them on their side

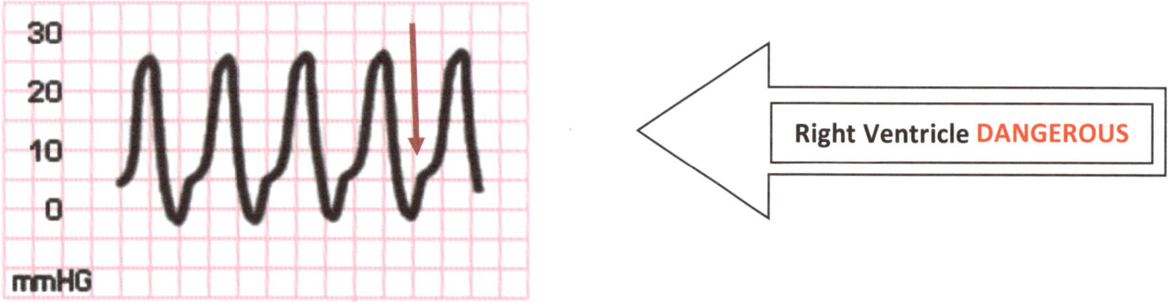

Pulmonary Artery Waveform

Pulmonary Artery Pressure **(PA)**

- 15-25mmHg systolic
- 8-15 mmHg diastolic
- Dicrotic notch on the right side
  - Referred to as a "high amplitude waveform"

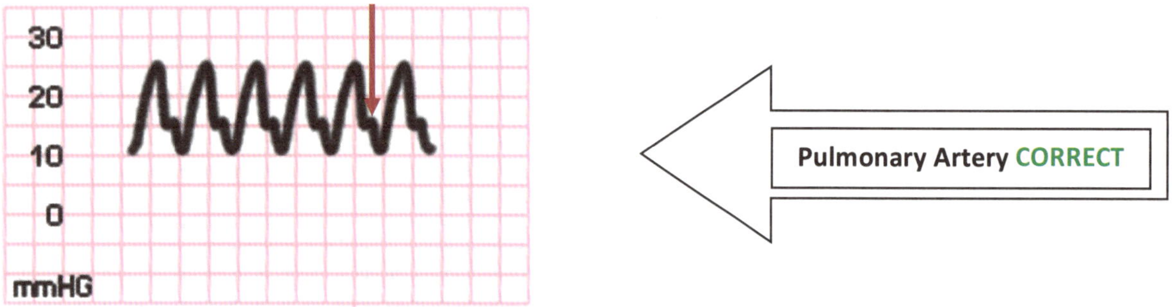

Causes of increased PA Pressures

- Left ventricular failure
- Liver failure (portal hypertension)
- Cor Pulmonale (increased pulmonary vascular resistance)
- Mitral Regurgitation
- Mitral Stenosis

"Wedge Waveform"

Pulmonary Artery Wedge Pressure (PAWP)

- Also called PACP (Pulmonary Artery Capillary Pressure) or PAOP (Pulmonary Artery Occlusion Pressure)
- These all represent the same pressure reading
- Wedge pressure = 8-12 mmHg (Left heart preload)
    - This waveform is caused by a blockage of the pulmonary artery by inflating the distal balloon. This is what allows the machine to get a "PAWP" (Pulmonary Artery Wedge Pressure)
- Referred to as a "low amplitude rolling waveform"

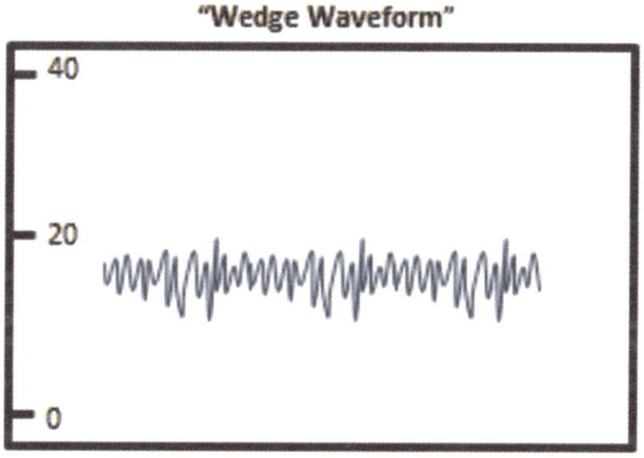

Cardiac Output Transducer

Utilizes a machine that is hooked up to the Swan-Ganz Catheter (this is not a separately inserted line)

- Placed at the phlebostatic axis (pictured below)
- 4th ICS, Mid Axillary Line

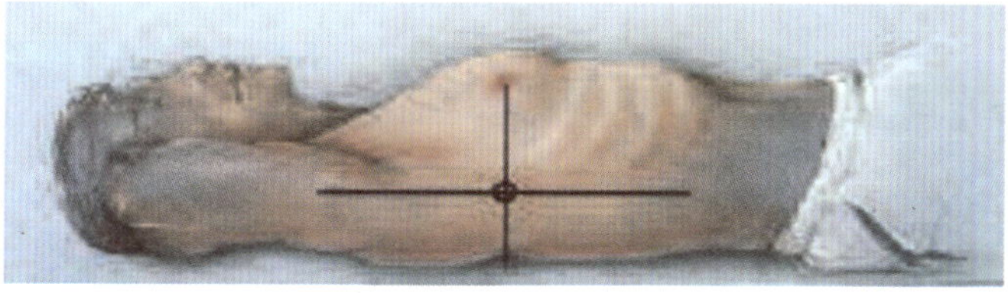

Overdamping- *system is not dynamic*

"Overdamping = Obstruction"

- Kinked line
- Obstruction in the tube

Underdamping- *system is too dynamic*

"Like having air in your brake lines"

- Pressure bag not full
- Air in the line

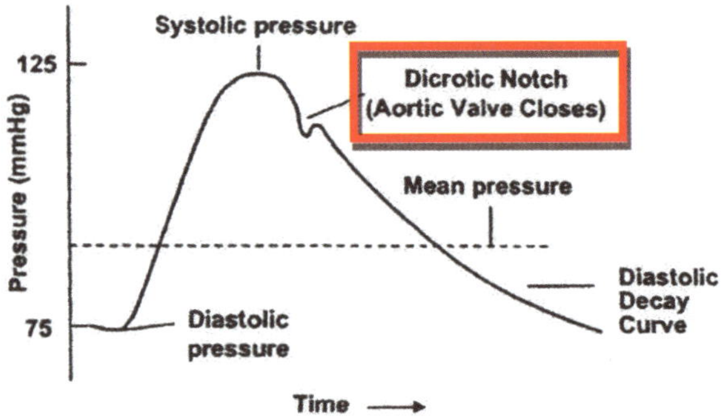

Intra-Aortic Balloon Pump (IABP)

Indications- Acute MI with cardiogenic shock, post coronary artery bypass graft (CABG)

Cardiogenic Shock

- Objective signs of shock due to heart failure
    - PAWP >18-20
    - ↓UOP
    - SBP <80mmHg

Contraindications- Aortic insufficiency/disease, severe peripheral vascular disease (PVD), or aortic regurgitation

- Can cause thrombocytopenia due to hemolysis (the balloon breaks some RBCs during inflation)

What the IABP does:

- ↑coronary perfusion
- ↓workload on heart

How the IABP functions

- Timed off of an EKG (can be manually adjusted)
  - Systole- Deflated
  - Diastole- Inflated

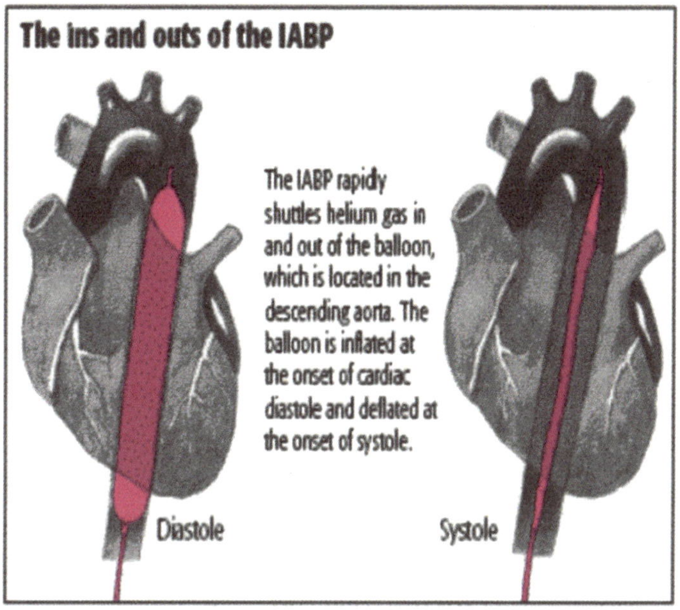

IABP Placement

- The IABP is directed towards the heart from the Femoral Artery
- Sits in the descending aorta, distal to Left Subclavian Artery, above Renal Artery
- Check placement by-
  - Checking LEFT radial pulse (left subclavian artery blockage causing limb ischemia)
  - Ensuring adequate UOP (Renal artery blockage which decreases UOP)
    Adult UOP is 0.5 ml/kg/hr *or* 30-50ml/hr
- CXR also confirms proper placement

IABP Pearls

- If there is a power failure, manually pump every 3-5 minutes to prevent blood from clotting on the balloon
- There is no need to purge IABP when going to altitude (the machine will purge itself)
- Ensure you carry extra helium tanks prior to transport (it is bad form to run out while in flight)
- If you see brown or rust colored flakes in IABP tubing, the tubing has ruptured (the brown flakes are clotted RBCs inside the tubing system

IABP Waveforms

"Normal" IABP Waveform

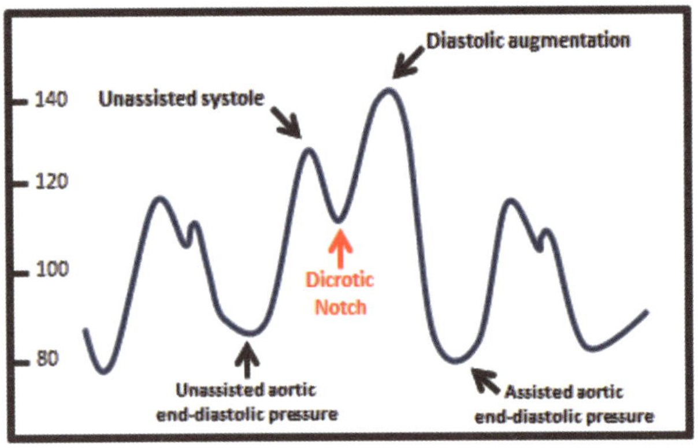

This is what the IABP waveform should look like
NORMAL

Late Deflation

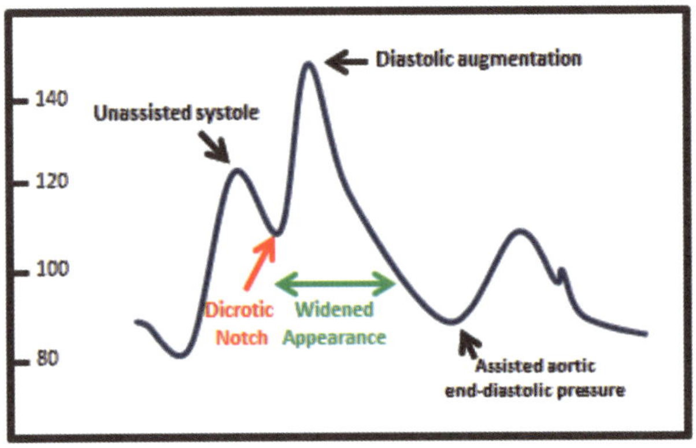

This is LATE deflation of the balloon pump
MOST DANGEROUS
↑Afterload

Late Deflation="Lethal Dose"

Early Inflation

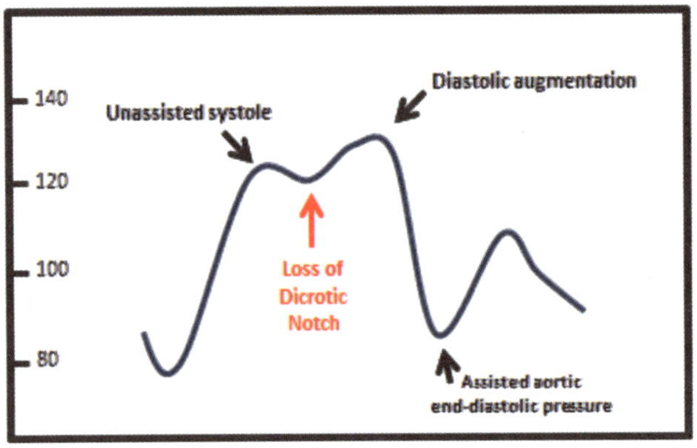

This is EARLY inflation of the balloon pump
DANGEROUS
Causes aortic regurgitation

Late Inflation

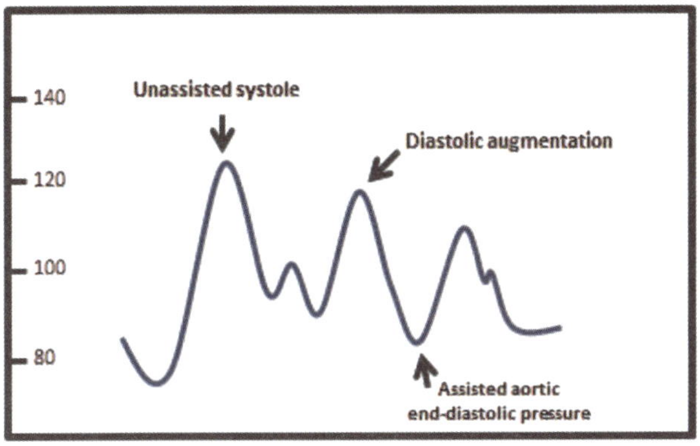

This is LATE inflation of the balloon pump
Sub-optimal coronary perfusion

Early Deflation

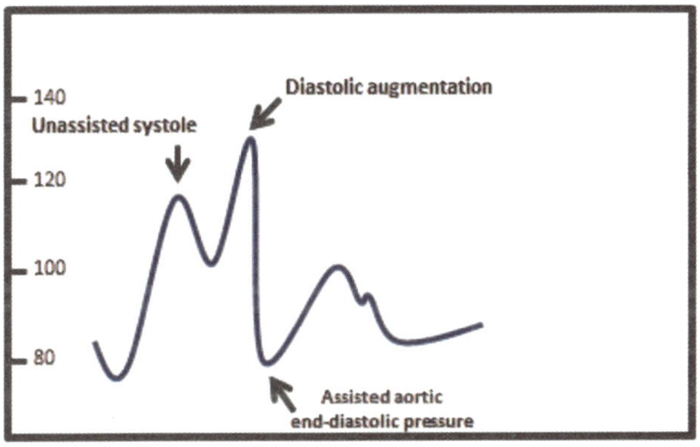

This is EARLY deflation of the balloon pump
Retrograde coronary blood flow

Obstetrical Emergencies (4)

Normal Maternal Changes

- HR increases 15-20 BPM
- B/P decreases 5-15 mmHg 2nd tri
  - B/P returns to "Normal" in 3rd tri
- Cardiac output increases
- Plasma increases 40%
  - Increase in clotting factors, increased risk of Pulmonary Embolus [PE]
- Hormones Progesterone and Relaxin relaxes sphincters
- Decreased functional / residual lung volume
  - Because the baby is taking up room in the belly

Pregnancy Terms

- Preterm- before 38 weeks
- Full term 38-42 weeks
- Post Term- after42 weeks

General Treatment Measures

- Place patient in the *right or left* lateral recumbent position
  - LLR (Left Lateral Recumbent) is preferred because it does not cause compression of the IVC (Inferior Vena Cava)
- Check temp (fever often indicates sepsis, give Ampicillin and Gentamycin [AMP+GENT])
- FHR (Fetal Heart Rate)
  - Normal FHR 120-160 BPM (Beats Per Minute)
- IV Lactated Ringers
- O_2

Assessment "DES"

- **D**ilation (0-10 cm)
- **E**ffacement (thickness of the cervix)
  - Normal is 2 CM
- **S**tation (fetal head in relation to the pubic bone (measured + or – in centimeters)

Fetal Monitoring

Internal Fetal monitoring

- Gold Standard- internal fetal monitoring (scalp transducer) with uterine pressure monitor (tocometer)
- Can use external fetal monitoring with Doppler

- Normal HR 120 to 160 BPM (baseline)
    - Fetal tachycardia is most commonly caused by maternal fever (sepsis)
    - Fetal bradycardia is most commonly caused by hypoxia

Variability

- The single most important predictor of fetal well being
- This is measured from beat to beat
- 10-15 bpm = normal variability
- #1 cause of poor variability- fetal hypoxia

Accelerations/Decelerations

- Are in relation to uterine contraction
- Example: early decel means the fetus' heart rate decelerates early in the uterine contraction cycle
- Accelerations are ALWAYS good
- *Decelerations can be bad*

Early Decelerations

- Mirrors contractions
- Associated with head pressed against the cervix
- *Benign*

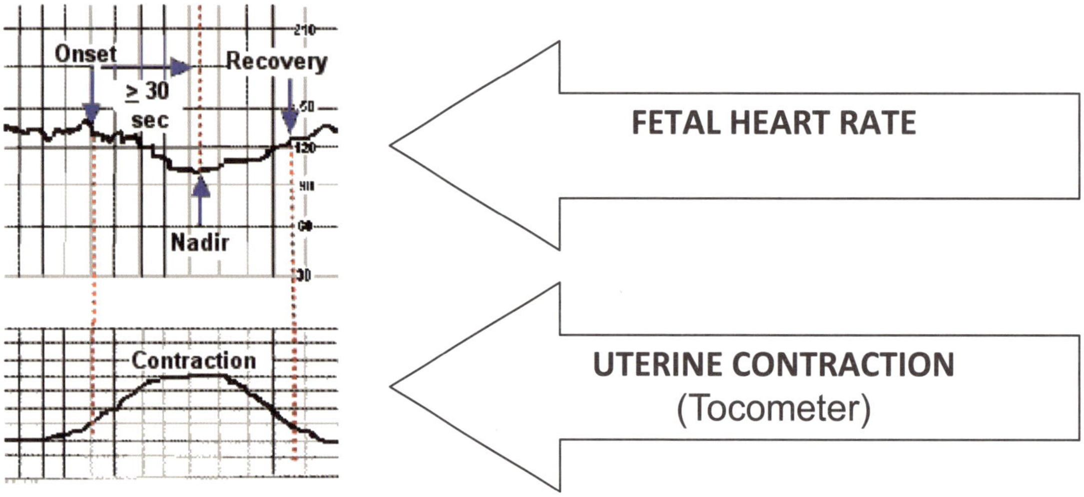

Late Decelerations

- Always indicates ureteroplacental insufficiency causing the fetus to experience a hypoxic bradycardia
- Commonly associated with PIH / DM / Smokers / Late Deliveries/ Pre Eclampsia
- Always concerning!

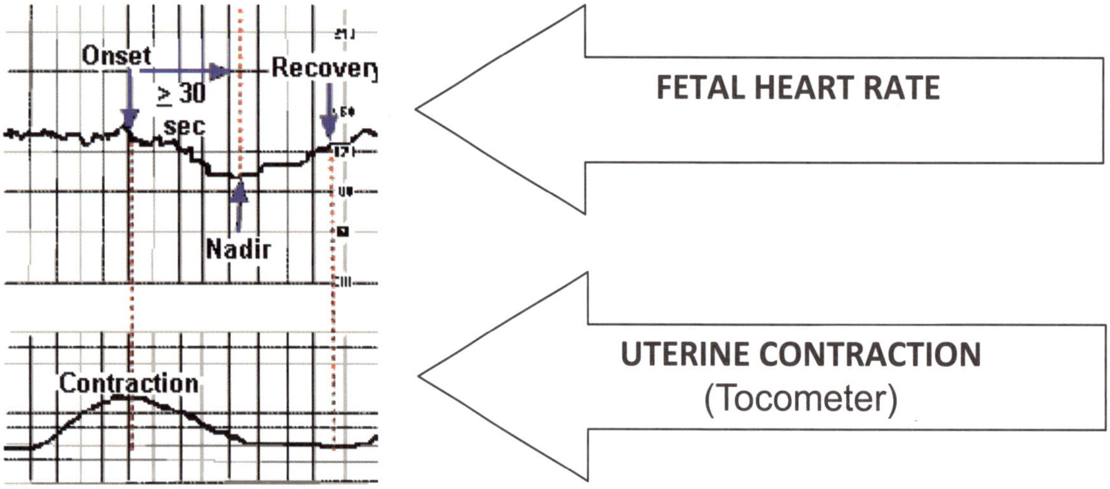

Variable Decelerations

- Caused by cord compression during uterine contraction

  Nucchal: Cord is wrapped around the fetus' neck

  - Clamp and cut cord if needed

  Prolapsed: Cord is protruding from the mother's vagina

  - Raise cord to relieve pressure, knees to chest, tocolytics, and saline gauze over exposed cord

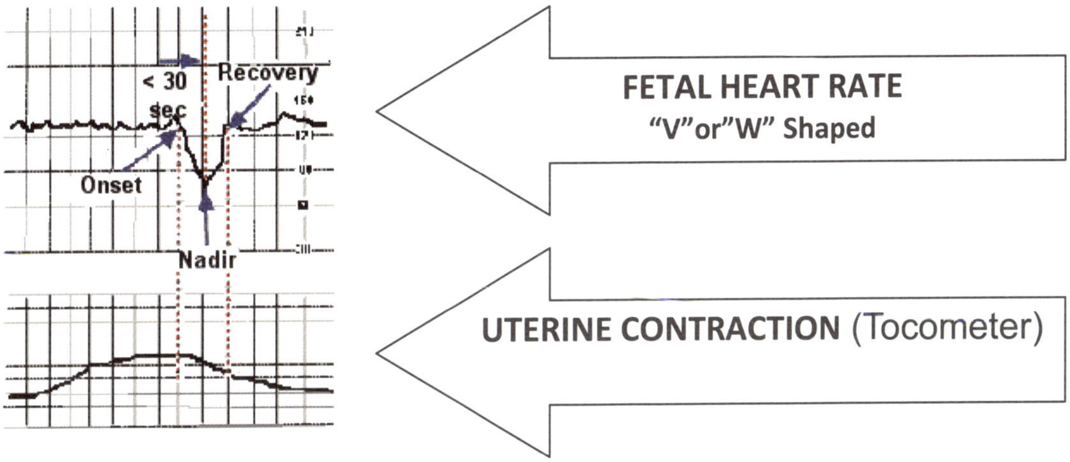

Sinusoidal Variations

- Caused by accidental tap of the umbilical cord during amniocentesis, fetomaternal transfusion, placental abruption
  - Fetal Hypovolemia
  - Anemia
  - Fetus is acidotic

- Emergency C-Section is indicated!

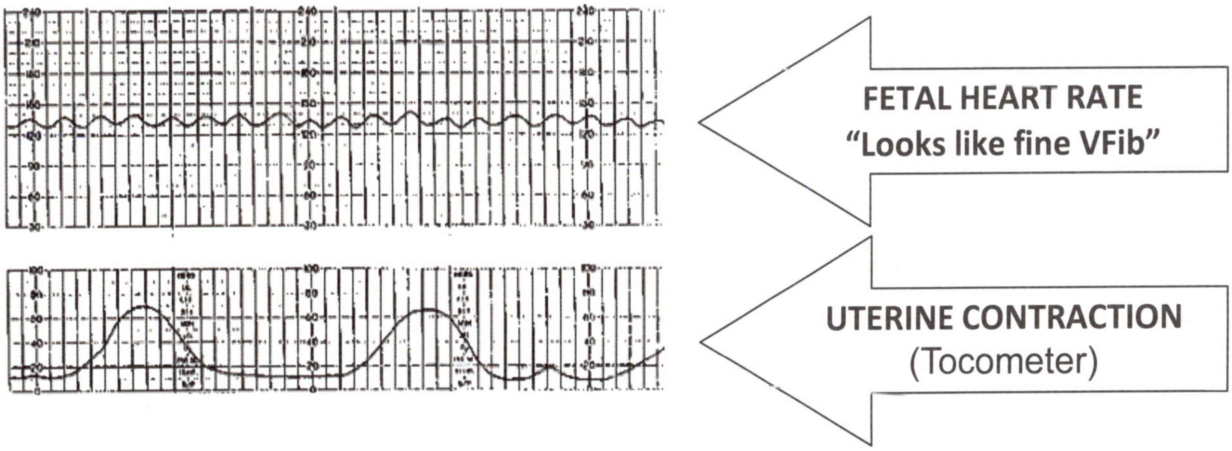

Signs of Imminent Delivery

- Vaginal bleeding (bloody show)
- Contractions < q10 min and increasing intensity
- Urge to push
- Need to have a BM
- Crowning

Stages of Delivery

1. Crowning (cervix is fully dilated)
2. Delivery of body
3. Delivery of placenta

Emergency C- Section Indications

- Multiple decelerations with poor rate / variability
- Sustained Bradycardia (<120 BPM for >10 minutes)
- Sinusoidal waveform

Delivery Complications

Pre-Term Labor

- Labor prior to 38 weeks gestation
- True labor presents with regular uterine contractions WITH cervical change (effacement)
    - Most common cause of preterm labor is Hypovolemia

Preterm Delivery

(<38 weeks)

Administer Tocolytics

- Terbutaline (fast acting, short half-life)
- Magnesium Sulfate (slower acting, long half-life)

Stimulate fetal lung maturity

- Steroids (Celestone, Dexamethasone)

Prevent infection

- Avoid vaginal examinations, if exam is needed use sterile gloves

Tocolytics

(Drugs that stop uterine contractions)

Terbutaline (Brethine)

- Stops tetanic contractions of the uterus IMMEDIATELY
  - *"Terbutaline for Tetany"*
- Subcutaneous 0.25mg q 15 min
- This is a *short* acting medication!
  - Think of it like Succinylcholine for RSI (works fast, but not for very long)

Magnesium Sulfate ("Mag")

- Mechanism of action- CNS depressant, smooth muscle relaxant
- Used to both prevent seizures in Pre-Eclampsia and as a tocolytic in pre-term labor
- Loading dose of 4-6 grams IV over 30 min
  - Continuous infusion rate of 2 grams/hour
- This is a *long* acting medication!
  - Think of it like Rocuronium for RSI (takes longer to work but lasts longer)
- Mag toxicity can occur, do a "Mag Check" to look for decreased DTRs, pulmonary edema
- The antidote for Magnesium Sulfate is Calcium Gluconate

"Mag Check"

- Deep Tendon Reflexes (DTRs)

  0: absent reflex

  1^+: trace, or seen only with reinforcement

  2^+: normal

  3^+: brisk

  4^+: nonsustained clonus (i.e., repetitive vibratory movements)

  5^+: sustained clonus
- Respirations (can cause pulmonary edema)
- DO NOT rely on blood levels of Mag, they do not correlate with levels of toxicity

Premature Rupture of Membranes

(PROM)

- This is found when a mother's "water breaks" and signifies that delivery is imminent
- If this occurs and the baby is preterm you must PREPARE FOR DELIVERY!
- The amniotic sac (membrane) surrounding the baby protects it from infection (sepsis)
- Administer steroids to stimulate fetal lung maturity!

Anaphylactoid Syndrome of Pregnancy

- Caused by maternal exposure to fetal cells, not an amniotic fluid PE [Pulmonary Embolus] as previously thought
    - ***DIC*** *(Disseminated Intravascular Coagulopathy)* ***and Anaphylaxis*** *at the same time*
- Symptoms- sudden onset of pleuritic chest pain, tachypnea, tachycardia, fever

Treatment

- Fluid resuscitation
- Increase PEEP (patient is hypoxic)
- Fresh Frozen Plasma(FFP), Platelets, Cryoprecipitate (Cryo)

Meconium

- Baby defecates while in the womb
    - Meconium is sterile (the baby has not eaten anything yet)
- Meconium inactivates surfactant
- Deep suction only if baby is not vigorous (strong cry, pink, active)
    - Intubate and suction below the vocal cords before the first cry

Umbilical Cord Prolapse

- Variable decelerations
- Elevate cord to relieve pressure (↑ fetal circulation)
    - Use saline soaked gauze to prevent the cord from drying (desiccation)
- Move to Trendelenburg position or knees to chest
    - Trendelenburg: feet 15 - 30 degrees above the head
- Give Tocolytics (Terbutaline, Mag Sulfate)

PIH

(Pregnancy Induced Hypertension)

- New onset hypertension (HTN) with pregnancy
- Can cause placental insufficiency
- Treatment options:
    - Labetolol (Beta Blocker)
    - Hydralazine (Alpresoline)
    - Methyldopa (Levodopa)

Shoulder Dystocia

- Shoulders will not pass through the pelvis
- Apply gentle traction to baby while applying suprapubic pressure

McRobert's maneuver

- Pulling the woman's knees towards her chest, applying suprapubic pressure

Turtle Sign: Appearance and retraction of the fetal head (like a turtle going back into it's shell)

Breech Delivery

- Don't touch until umbilicus is delivered
- Don't attempt a footling breech

Mauriceau's maneuver

- Fingers relieving pressure off the baby's nose so they can breath
- Downward suprapubic pressure while the baby is rotated out of the birth canal

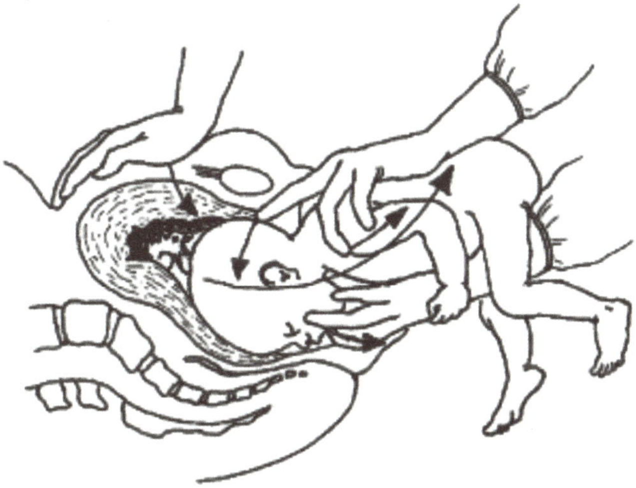

HELLP Syndrome

(Hemolysis / Elevated Liver Enzymes / Low Platelets)

- Commonly seen with PreEclampsia and Eclampsia
- RUQ pain (liver), jaundice, malaise
- Give Mag Sulfate (4-6 G over 30 minutes)
- Steroids (Celestone or Dexamethasone) to stimulate fetal lung maturity
- Hypertension- use Labetalol, Hydralazine, or Methyldopa

***Pre*Eclampsia**

- HTN/ Proteinuria/Edema
- *NO SEIZURES*
- Risk factors- extremes of age, 1st pregnancy
- Often causes LATE DECELERATIONS

Eclampsia

- HTN/ Proteinuria/Edema
- *GENERALIZED SEIZURES*
- Seizures are treated with valium
- Give Mag Sulfate to depress seizure activity
    - Sign of Mag toxicity is ↓ DTRs (*hyporeflexia), pulmonary edema*
    - Antidote for Mag Sulfate toxicity is Calcium Gluconate
- Note: Benzos are usually contraindicated in pregnancy; they are only indicated in the treatment of seizures in pregnancy

Maternal Hemorrhage

Placenta Abruption

EMERGENCY

- *Painful* bleeding
- Any MVA or blunt trauma is placental abruption until proven otherwise
- Causes exsanguination & placental insufficiency

Placenta Previa

Not an emergency (unless there is hemorrhage)

- *Painless* bright red bleeding
- DO NOT DISTURB THE VAGINA!
    - Avoid any vaginal exams

Postpartum Hemorrhage (PPH)

- >500 ml blood loss (anytime within 24 hours after delivery)
- First line treatment is vigorous fundal massage!
    - Bimanual uterine compression

Pitocin

- Drug that causes contraction of the uterus to help stop bleeding

Methergine

- Drug that causes contraction of the uterus to help stop bleeding

Oxytocin

- Released by the pituitary in large amounts;
    - After distension of the cervix and uterus during labor, facilitating birth
    - After stimulation of the nipples
    - During breastfeeding
        - This is one reason why babies are placed on mothers chest after birth

Pitocin
(Synthetic Oxytocin)

- Often used for uterine atony after placental delivery in the setting of continued maternal hemorrhage

Uterine Rupture

- "Stomach is as hard as a board"
    - Caused by peritonitis
- "Fetal parts presenting under the mother's skin"

- #1 cause of maternal death is trauma
- #1 cause of fetal death is maternal death

Rh Negative Mothers

- Rhogam prevents mothers immune response to the baby's Rh positive cells (prevents mom's immune system from attacking the baby).

- If a mother is Rh negative, ALWAYS give Rhogam!
    - This means the mother has Rh antibodies
    - The majority of the population is Rh positive

- When to give Rhogam-
    - At 28 weeks gestation
    - After delivery
    - After ANY trauma/bleeding/potential bleeding

Miscellaneous OB Pearls

- Do not pull on the umbilical cord after delivery of the baby, this can cause uterine inversion
    - Uterine inversion requires manual replacement

- Gestational diabetic mothers are more likely to give birth to children with hypoglycemia
    - The neonate is typically larger than normal (fetal macrosomia)
    - This is because the baby's pancreas produces insulin at normal levels, and once no longer inside the mother the glucose levels drop dramatically
    - HYPOGLYCEMIA IS A COMMON CAUSE OF SEIZURES IN THE NEWBORN

Condition	Treatment
Hypertension	Labetolol, Hydralazine, Methyldopa
Post-Partum Hemorrhage	Fundal Massage, Pitocin, Methergine
Seizures	Valium
Uterine Contractions	Terbutaline, Mag Sulfate
PreEclampsia/Eclampsia	Mag Sulfate

Neonatal Emergencies (4)
(Birth to 28 days old)

Neonatal Airway

- Infant heads are larger in proportion to the rest of the body
    - Results in a natural sniffing position
- Neonates and infants are obligate nasal breathers
    - Suction the mouth first, then the nose (Stimulating the nares first may cause gasping)
    - Can use a bulb syringe, DeLee Suction, or 10F or 14F suction catheter
- Airway secretion and edema can cause serious problems earlier than in adults
- Consider nasogastric tubes in all intubated neonates

Meconium

- Meconium is sterile (consists of hair, teeth, skin cells, etc)
- Deep suction (below the vocal cords) is ONLY indicated if the neonate is not vigorous if meconium is present at birth
- Surfactant is inactivated by meconium

Isolette™ (Incubator)

- Device to put any preterm or term infant into to maintain heat, provide supplemental oxygen, and to protect from the environment. (Isolette™ is a brand name)
- Commonly used for preterm infant
- Indications:
    - Preterm neonate <5 kg
    - Distress in a baby less than 28 days from date of birth (neonate)
- Infants and Peds lose heat quicker than adults because of their large body surface area to mass index ratio
- Patient must be secured inside the incubator during flight

Neonatal Infectious Disease

- Top 3 killers in the first 24 hours
    - Sepsis
    - Respiratory complications
    - Cardiac problems

Neonatal Sepsis

- Most commonly caused by Group B Strep
- Occurs in utero –often caused by **P**remature **R**upture **O**f **M**embranes (PROM)
- Treatment: Ampicillin + Gentamycin (Amp + Gent)

Infant Seizures

- Infant Seizures- S/Sx include lip smacking and tongue thrusting, eye fluttering, lowered O_2 sats
    - "Subtle Seizures"
- Common causes:
    - Hypoglycemia
    - Opiod withdrawal
    - Interventricular hemorrhage (preterm infant bleeding inside the ventricles of the brain)

Febrile Seizures

- Rate of temperature increase is the most important factor (not overall temp)
- Fever- Each 1° change >37° HR increases 10 BPM
- Does not require further workup if the cause is known (ear infection, viral illness, etc.)

Choanal Atresia

- A congenital disorder where the back of the nasal passage (choana) is blocked, usually by abnormal bony or soft tissue formed during fetal development
- Remember that Infants are obligate nasal breathers for the first 6 months
- Likely will require intubation

Respiratory Distress Syndrome (RDS)

(Also called Hyaline Membrane Disease "HMD")

- Surfactant deficiency
- Surfactant reduces surface tension in the alveoli
- Newborn has increased work of breathing, tachypnea
- #1 killer of premature infants (born <38 Weeks)
- Consider use of surfactant when transporting preterm infants (given via ETT)

Persistent Pulmonary Hypertension of the Newborn

"PPHN"

- *Right to Left Shunt*
- Characterized by marked pulmonary hypertension that causes hypoxia
- Likely will have a patent foramen ovale and patent ductus arteriosus
- Consider surfactant (given via ETT)

Omphalocele

"O" Abdominal ring, protrusion of viscera (arrest of development of the abdominal wall)

- Is attached to the umbilical cord
- This condition is WORSE than Gastroschesis (high morbidity)
- Treat like an abdominal evisceration!
    - Maintain body temperature
    - Cover with moist, sterile dressings
    - Keep NPO
    - Will require surgical repair

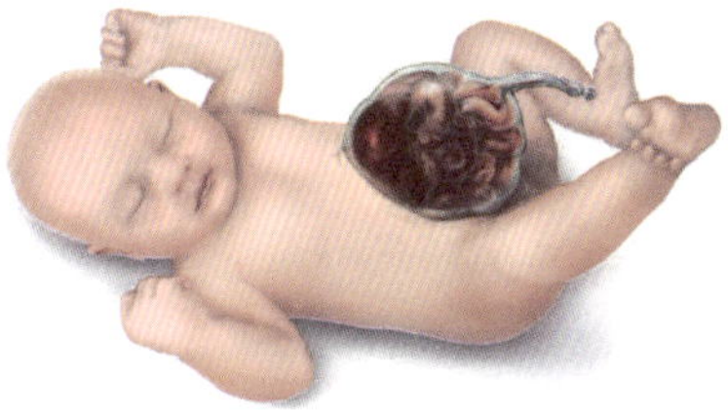

GASTROSCHESIS

Defect with completed development of internal organs. Abdominal contents are coming out of the body on one side of the umbilical cord.

- Treat like an abdominal evisceration!
    - Maintain body temperature
    - Cover with moist, sterile dressings
    - Keep NPO
    - Will require surgical repair
- This is less severe than an Omphalocele!

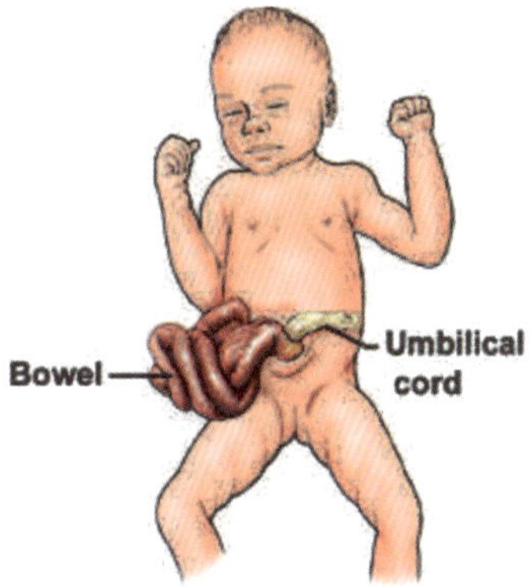

Ventriculoperitoneal Shunt

"VP Shunt"

- Treatment for increased CSF in congenital hydrocephalus ("water in the brain")
- Cerebral spinal fluid can build up leading to an increase in intracranial pressure (ICP)
- Intracranial hematoma
- Cerebral edema
- Brainstem herniation
- Patient often presents with gastric distention, mental status changes, ↓LOC, vomiting, seizures
  - Give Mannitol
  - Raise the head of the bead 30° (Semi-Fowlers)

Shaken Baby Syndrome

- Causes a diffuse axonal injury (DAI)
  - Bulging fontanelles
  - Increased ICP
  - Retinal hemorrhages

Neonatal Cardiac Problems

- Newborns with a HR ≤60 and a D-Stick ≤60:
  - *Administer Epinephrine 1st* (1:10,000) 0.1 to 0.3 ml/kg by IV or ETT
    - Do not use the 1:1000 concentration in newborns
  - *Then Glucose (2cc/kg D10)*
- Cardiomegaly + Hepatomegaly (enlarged heart and liver) means the child has CHF (congestive heart failure)
  - Stop IV Fluids, administer Digitalis
- Worsening cyanosis in a crying infant indicates a cardiac problem
- Most common cardiac defect is a Ventricular Septal Defect (VSD), a hole between the ventricles

Patent Ductus Arteriosis

(PDA)

- This is a blood vessel connecting the pulmonary artery to the aortic arch. It allows most of the blood from the right ventricle to bypass the fetus's fluid-filled non-functioning lungs
- Upon closure at birth, it becomes the ligamentum arteriosum
- PGE1 (Prostaglandin E1) is what keeps the PDA open (PGE1 administration can cause apnea)
- Indocin (Indomethacin) is the drug of choice for closing a PDA
  - Oxygen also closes the PDA
- Cyanotic lesions are often PDA dependent (DO NOT CLOSE THE PDA)
- PDA problems are often found on physical exam by checking for femoral pulses
- If femoral pulses are absent, possible coarctation of the aorta, patient likely requires PDA to survive

Tetralogy of Fallot

- *Right to Left Shunt*

Consists of the following defects:

- Pulmonary Stenosis
- Aortic Coarctation
- Transposition of Great Vessels (the aorta and pulmonary arteries are switched)
- Ventricular Septal Defect (VSD)

- "Tet Spells" are characterized by sudden cyanosis and syncope
- Treat with knees to chest, Morphine
- If knees to chest/morphine does not resolve "tet spell" perform RSI, intubate, 100% O2

Miscellaneous Neonates

- An umbilical cord normally has 2 arteries and 1 vein
- If the newborn only has 1 artery and 1 vein in the cord (referred to as a "single artery cord"), the Renal system is likely to be affected

Pediatric Emergencies (10)

Age Ranges

Classification	Age
Neonate	Birth to 28 days
Infant	28 days to 1 year old
Toddler	1 year old to 2 years old
Child	>2 years old

Emergency Intervention Formulas

ETT Diameter $\frac{(16+Age)}{4}$

- If the required ETT size is ≥5.5mm a CUFFED ETT should be used. If < 5.5 use an UNCUFFED ETT
- Cricothyroidotomy only if >11 y/o

"2/3/4 Rule"

2 x ETT Size = Suction/NG Foley diameter (ex. 5.0 ETT = 10fr Foley)

3 x ETT Size = ETT Insertion depth (ex. 7.0 ETT = 21cm insertion depth)

4 x ETT Size = Chest Tube (ex. 5.0 ETT = 20fr chest tube)

NOTES: If the ETT size required for a child is >5.5 mm use a cuffed ETT!
Once intubation is complete, place a Nasogastric Tube (NG Tube) to decompress the stomach

Normal Systolic B/P $90 + (2\ x\ Age)$

Hypotensive Systolic B/P $70 + (2\ x\ Age)$

Defibrillation 2J/kg

Pediatric Fluid Resuscitation

Emergency

Neonate / Infant 10cc/kg (<1 year old)

Toddler/Child 20cc/kg (>1 year old)

*Do not give more than 2 bolus infusions

Average Circulating blood volume in a child = 80-90 ml/kg

Pediatric Maintenance Fluids "4/2/1"

Non-Emergency

1-10 kg → 4cc/kg/hr
10-20 kg → 2cc/kg/hr
>20 kg → 1cc/kg/hr

Example: A 25 kg child needs fluids. First 10kg= 40cc, second 10kg = 20cc, last 5kg = 5cc
Answer: total fluid required= 65cc/hr

- *THESE RATES ARE cc PER HOUR!* *(cc and mL are the same thing)*

Pediatric Glucose Management

D stick <60mg/dL

Neonate	2cc/kg D10
Infant/Toddler	2cc/kg D25
Child	2cc/kg D50

Pediatric Airway Problems

- Stridor- Inhalation problem
  - involves the *upper* airway
- Wheezing- Exhalation problem
  - involves the *lower* airway

Bronchiolitis

(Swelling of the bronchiole walls) ***Usually not life threatening***

- >90% viral
- Cough, shortness of breath, nasal flaring, wheezing/crackling on exam
- Often caused by RSV (Respiratory Syncytial Virus)
- Isolation required (highly contagious)
- Treatment: Supportive care, O_2, Fluids, Isolation
- Watch for apnea!

Croup

(Swelling around the vocal cords) ***Usually not life threatening***

- *Gradual onset* with URI, no drooling
- "Seal Like" barking cough
- **Steeple Sign** on A/P neck x-ray
  - "The crow lives in the steeple"
- Treat with racemic epinephrine and steroids (Decadron)
  - Racemic epinephrine is used because it is nebulized (aerosolized)

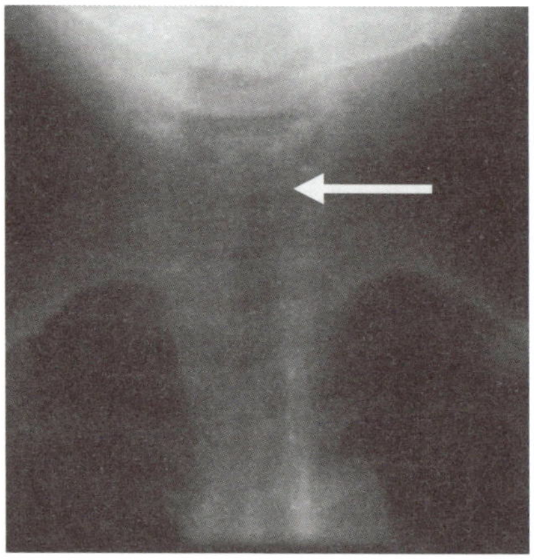

Epiglottitis

(Swelling of the epiglottis) **LIFE THREATENING**

- *Sudden onset, DROOLING*
- Patient presents in the "tripod position"
- **Thumb sign** on lateral neck x ray (looks like a thumbprint)
- **Do not disturb the child due to possible rapid airway loss**
- Treatment: Antibiotics, humidified O_2

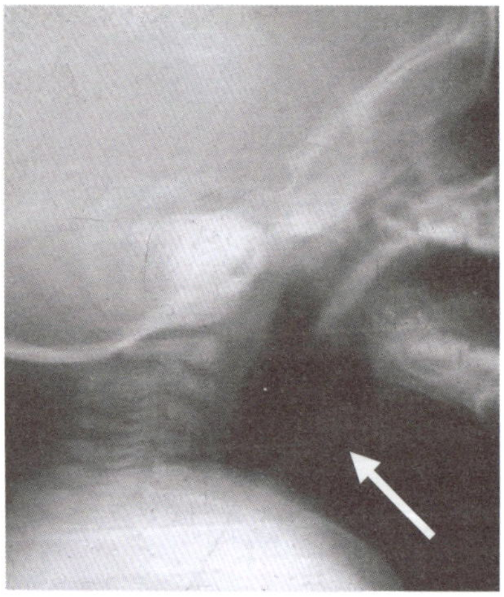

Respiratory Syncytial Virus (RSV)

- Lower respiratory tract infection
    - RSV CAN CAUSE APNEA!
- More common in those with:
    - Congenital heart defect (CHD)
    - Hyaline Membrane Disease (HMD)
    - Bronchopulmonary dysplasia (BPD)
- Treatment is limited to supportive care and oxygen therapy.

Pediatric Trauma

Waddel's Triad Δ (child hit by a car)

1) Car hits them
2) They hit the car
3) They hit the ground

- When falling, children strike their heads first
- Most common cause of traumatic death in Peds is Motor Vehicle Accidents
- Most commonly organ injured is the skin
- Children do not show signs of hypotension until >25% blood loss (they compensate with tachycardia)

Accidental Ingestion

- Narcotics- Decreased respiratory drive and altered mental status
- If unknown cause of ingestion, give Narcan and Flumazenil
- All other agents, give supportive care (Airway, IV, O_2)

Pediatric Abuse

- Multiple fractures or bruises in different stages of healing
- Retinal hemorrhages

Misc. Peds bullets:

- Peds are belly breathers
    - Infants are obligate nasal breathers
- Bradycardia/Cardiac Arrest is most commonly secondary to hypoxia
- The most narrow portion of the pediatric airway is the cricoid ring in children <10 y/o
- A child's primary emotion is fear

Neurological Emergencies (10)

MAP (Mean Arterial Pressure) $= \frac{SBP + (2 \times DBP)}{3}$ Normal 80 to 100 mmHg (ideally 90mmHg)

CPP (Cerebral Perfusion Pressure) = MAP - ICP Normal 60-80 mmHg (Keep above 60mmHg)

ICP normal value 0 – 10 mmHg ICP > 20mmHg has high mortality (Monroe-Kellie Doctrine)

ICP Transducer is placed at the foramen of Monro (level of the ear)

Signs/Sx of Herniation

- Change in LOC
- Pupil reaction
- Decorticate/Decerebrate posturing
    - Decorticate "to the core", associated with brainstem herniation

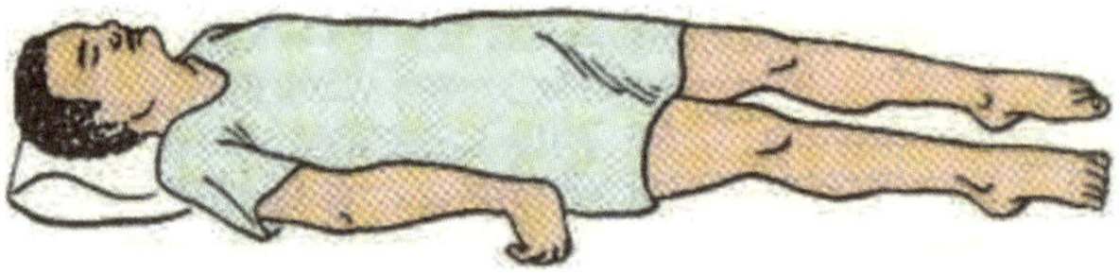

A. Extension posturing (decerebrate rigidity)

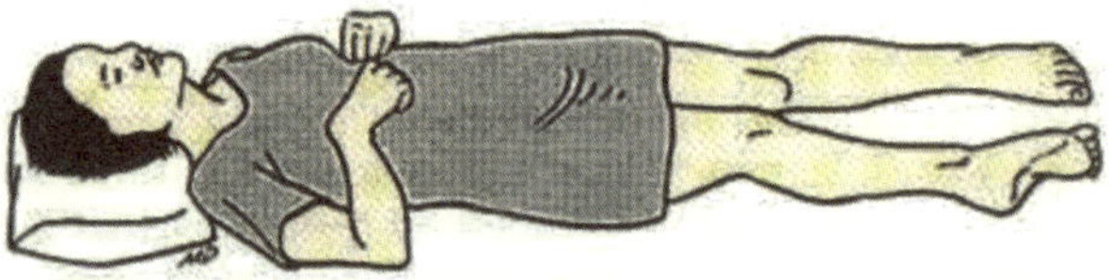

B. Abnormal flexion (decorticate rigidity)

Cushing's Triad Δ- results from increased ICP leading to brainstem herniation

- Hypertension
- Bradycardia
- Increased Pulse Pressure (Systolic and diastolic numbers are far apart, ex 180/60)

Respiratory Changes

- Cheyne-Stokes: breathing becoming shallower until it stops for a while (apnea) and then breathing starts again and rapidly crescendos to a peak before decreasing away

Cheyne-Stoke's Respirations

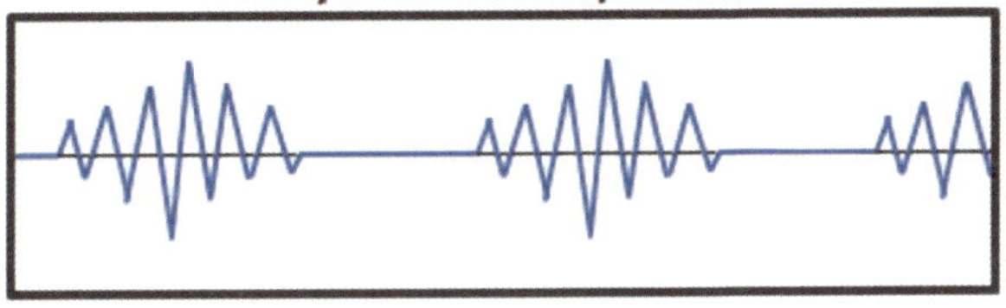

- Depending on the text you read Cushing's Δ includes either widened pulse pressure or repiratory changes. This is not clinically significant or significant for the exam

Treatment of Brainstem Herniation

• Paralyze	(RSI)
• Intubate	(RSI)
• Hyperventilate	(Goal $PaCO_2$ 30-35mmHg)
• Mannitol	(Decrease fluid in the cranial vault, 1g/kg IV bolus over 5 min)
• Hypertonic Saline	(Give slowly to prevent Central Pontine Myelinolysis)
• Barbiturate Coma	(Lowers O_2 demand)

Hypoxia and Hypercapnia cause cerebral blood vessels to dilate, increasing blood flow and volume, further escalating ICP

Treat seizures with a Benzo, and then give either Phenytoin (Dilantin) or Fosphenytoin (Cerberyx)

- Dilantin : 1G loading dose infused at 50mg/min

Lasix can be used in the setting of herniation AFTER Mannitol (it won't work as well as Mannitol though)

Central Pontine Myelinolysis is caused by reversing hyponatremia (low sodium) too quickly. It causes the brain to shrink like a raisin.

DO NOT USE HYPOTONIC SOLUTIONS OR GLUCOSE!

- Hyponatremia is associated with brain edema
- Hyperglycemia makes brain injuries worse

Skull Fractures

Diastatic Fracture: along the suture lines of the skull, leads to a separation of the sutures

Linear Fracture: extends towards the base of the skull

- Associated with Epidural Hematoma and infection
    - Dirt and hair getting in the opening into the cranial vault

Linear Stellate Fracture: multiple fractures that radiate form the compressed area

- Spider web appearance

Basilar Skull Fracture–results from an extension of fractures from the calvaria (roof of the skull)

- Battle's Sign, Raccoon Eyes, Otorrhea, clear rhinorrhea (CSF leak), hemotympanum (blood behind TM)
- NO Nasotracheal intubation, Nasopharyngeal airways, Nasogastric tubes

Orbital Fracture- a fracture of the orbital rim (eye socket) that is caused by a direct blow

- Potentially serious complication of the inferior rectus eye muscle becoming trapped
- Have the patient look up, if one eye doesn't go up (and causes double vision) it is a surgical emergency

Depressed Skull Fracture- caused by a blow to the head (usually with a hammer or something similar)

- Can lead to a Pneumocephalus (air trapped inside the skull) if any of the sinus cavities are fractured
- Pneumocephalous can become worse when going to altitude causing brainstem herniation
    - Trapped air expands due to Boyle's law

Head injuries are the leading cause of death in the trauma victim!

Concussions

- Mild - knocked out, no memory loss
- Classic – Memory loss
- Diffuse Axonal injury – Coma

Glasgow Coma Scale

Eye Opening	
Spontaneous	4
To Loud Voice	3
To Pain	2
None	1

Verbal Response	
Oriented	5
Confused, Disoriented	4
Innapropriate Words	3
Incomprehensible Sounds	2
None	1

Best Motor Response	
Obeys	6
Localizes	5
Withdraws (Flexion)	4
Abnormal flexion Posturing	3
Extension Posturing	2
None	1

Minor Injury 13 – 15
Moderate Injury 9 – 12
Severe Injury <8

Hypertensive Urgency/Emergency

Hypertensive Urgency

- Condition where a patient has extremely elevated blood pressure with NO signs or symptoms of end organ damage
- Blood pressure should be lowered slowly
- Not an emergency (yet)

Hypertensive Crisis/Emergency-

- Condition where a patient has extremely elevated blood pressure WITH signs and symptoms of end organ damage
    - Headache, Nausea/Vomiting, Visual Changes
    - Creatinine/RBCs in Urine

Treatment:

- Lower B/P no more than 25% per hour, and no lower than patients "normal" pressure
    - Use Labetolol and Nitroprusside (Nipride)

Cerebral Bleeding

Subdural Hematoma **(SDH)** **"Venous Lakes"**

- Results from a tearing of the bridging veins to the subdural space
- This has a slow onset (over several hours)
- Often in the elderly, kids
- More common and more lethal than epidural hematomas
    - Interventricular hemorrhage has increased mortality

Epidural Hematoma **"MMA"**

- Arterial bleed, M/C vessel damaged is the middle meningeal artery "MMA"
- LOC followed by a lucid interval (being awake) and an second LOC
- Example: football player unconscious for a minute, wakes up, then goes unconscious 30 minutes later
- Pupil dilation after occulomotor nerve injury due to loss of parasympathetic tone
- Cheyne-Stokes Respirations common

Subarachnoid Hemorrhage (SAH) **"Worst headache of my life"**

- This is a LIFE THREATENING cause of headache
- Starfish Pattern on CT, Xanthochromia on lumbar puncture (blood tinged CSF)
- Avoid lumbar punctures until CT Scan complete
- Keep systolic B/P below 140mmHg
- Treat with Nimodepine (Nimotop)
    - Helps prevent cerebral vasospasm
- Patients with persistent elevated B/P in the setting of intracranial hemorrhage should be treated with Nitroprusside (Nipride)

Miscellaneous

- Important dermatomes: T4 nipples, T10 umbilicus, C3/4/5 innervates the diaphragm

Autonomic Dysreflexia

"Autonomic Hypereflexia"

- Common occurrence in the paralyzed patient that does not have a Foley in place
    - The bladder becomes extremely distended
    - Common in spinal cord injuries
- Increases B/P, H/R, ICP
- Insert and drain a Foley catheter slowly

Spinal Cord Injuries

Babinski's Sign (reflex): Occurs when the big toe moves toward the top surface of the foot and the other toes fan out after the sole of the foot has been firmly stroked

- Important physical exam finding in spinal cord injuries

- Spinal cord injuries at or above the C5 level result in apnea or bradypnea (decreased respirations)
- C3/4/5 "Keeps the diaphragm alive"

Brown Sequard Lesion

- Ipsilateral motor & vibratory sense loss below the level of injury
    - Ipsilateral = Same side
- Contralateral pain & temperature loss
    - Contralateral = Opposite side

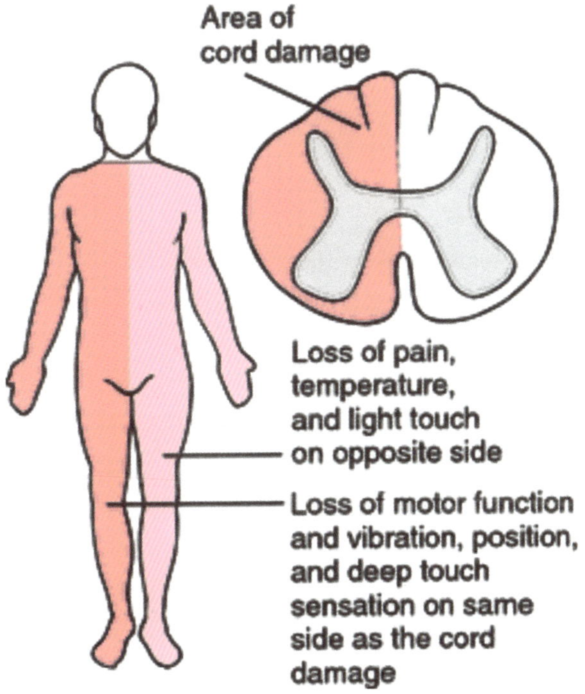

Central Cord injury

- Motor weakness in upper extremities (UE) is greater than lower extremities (LE)
    - This is below the level of injury
- UE>LE

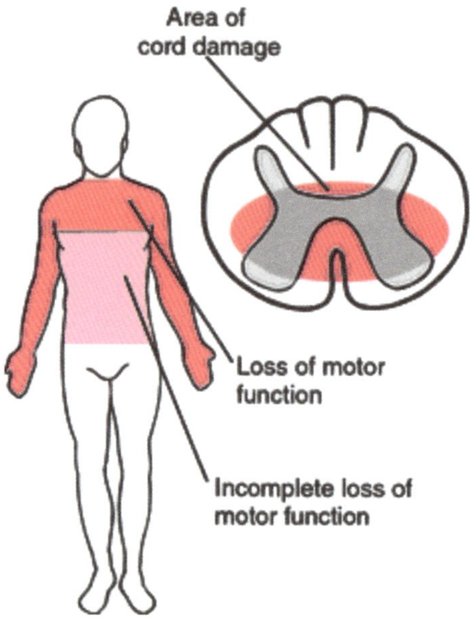

Anterior Cord Syndrome

- Loss of pain & temperature sensation everywhere below the level of injury
- Sparing of proprioreception & vibration
- WORST PROGNOSIS

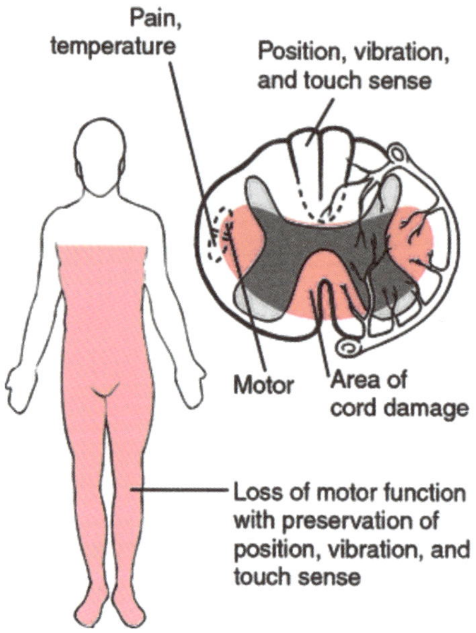

Spinal Shock

- Due to swelling of the spinal cord after trauma
- Decreased Systemic Vascular Resistance (SVR)
    - SVR <800
- Hypotension
- Treat with IV fluids & vasopressors
- Can treat with high dose steroids (controversial)

Neurogenic Shock
(Distributive Shock)

- Causes a decrease in sympathetic nervous system outflow
    - Unable to vasoconstrict and increase HR
- Occurs due to spinal cord swelling after trauma
- Decreased Systemic Vascular Resistance (SVR) and normal heart rate
    - SVR <800
- Hypotension
- Warm red skin
- No tachycardia
- Treat with IV fluids & Vasopressors

Meningitis

- Caused by inflammation of the meninges
- Disease is carried in the Cerebral Spinal Fluid (CSF)
- Treatment is based on cause (bacterial, viral, fungal, etc.)
- Triad of nuchal rigidity (neck stiffness), photophobia (intolerance of bright light) and headache

Brudzinki's Sign: the appearance of involuntary lifting of the legs when lifting a patient's head with the patient lying supine

Kernig's Sign: Severe stiffness of the hamstrings causes an inability to straighten the leg when the hip is flexed to 90 degrees ("Kicking Kernigs")

Use personal protective measures

- Gloves
- Mask
- Gown

Cerebro Vascular Accident (CVA)

"Brain Attack"

- Keep stroke patients slightly hypertensive to maintain Cerebral Perfusion Pressure (CPP)

Neuroprotective Agents

- Currently, the only approved medical therapy for acute ischemic stroke is tissue plasminogen activator (tPA), a thrombolytic agent that targets the thrombus within the blood vessel

- IV (Intravenous) TPA if <3 hrs from incident
- IA (Intrarterial) TPA <6hrs (medication pushed directly into the clot)
- MERCI if 8 to 12 hrs old (roto-rooter)

Herpes Simplex Encephalitis

- Most common cause of encephalitis in the U.S.
- Caused by Herpes Simplex Virus (HSV) type 1 (the one that causes cold sores)
- Patient often has fever, seizures, headache, decreased LOC, and focal neurologic defecit
- Treat HSV with IV Acyclovir

Seizures

Generalized Seizures

Absence seizures are an abrupt and sudden onset impairment of consciousness, interruption of ongoing activities, a blank stare

Atonic (drop seizures or drop attacks) are a brief lapse in muscle tone that are caused by temporary alterations in brain function. The seizures are brief - usually less than fifteen seconds

Tonic-Clonic (grand mal seizures) are a type of generalized seizure that affects the entire brain. Tonic–clonic seizures are the seizure type most commonly associated with epilepsy and seizures in general

Myoclonic involve brief, involuntary twitching of a muscle or a group of muscles

Partial Seizures (also called focal or localized seizures)

Simple Partial seizures have preserved consciousness while experiencing of unusual feelings or sensations, and usually the event is remembered in detail

Complex Partial can have automatisms such as lip smacking, chewing or swallowing (also called "subtle seizures)

Status Epilepticus is one continuous, unremitting seizure lasting longer than 30 minutes or recurrent seizures without regaining consciousness between seizures for greater than 30 minutes

Lab Studies you MUST know

ABGs (Arterial Blood Gasses)

pH 7.35 – 7.45 (percentage of Hydrogen ions)

[technically pH is an inverse log of hydrogen ions]

CO_2 35-45 (Carbon Dioxide)

[this is the respiratory component of an ABG, and is acidic]

HCO_3 22-26 (Bicarbonate)

[this is the metabolic component of an ABG, and is alkalotic or "basic"]

PaO_2 80-100 mmHg (Plasma pressure concentration of Oxygen)

PaO_2 Levels	SaO_2 Levels (pulse ox)
90 mmHg	100%
60 mmHg	90%
30 mmHg	60%
27 mmHg	50%

SaO_2 > 95% (Hemoglobin saturation of Oxygen)

[this is the same measurement that a "pulse ox" gives]

BE -2 to 2 (Base Excess)

[a base deficit of ≥ -4 is an indicator for potential need for blood transfusion]

[a base deficit of ≥-19 correlates with a poor outcome {death likely}]

Replacement Formula: 0.1 x (-BE) x patient weight in kg = Bicarb needed

Example: Patient weighs 100kg and has a BE of -5. Formula 0.1 x (-5) x 100kg = 50 meq Bicarb required

ABG	Normal Range
pH	7.35 - 7.45
CO_2	35 - 45
HCO_3	22 - 26
PaO_2	80-100
SaO_2	> 95%
Base (Deficit/Excess)	(-2) to (2+)

ABG Interpretation

1. Is the pH Acidotic (<7.35) or Alkalotic (>7.45)?

   a. CO_2 (Carbon Dioxide) is an Acid, so more CO_2 makes the ABG more acidotic (moves left)

      - *Technically CO_2 is not an acid. CO_2 combines with H_2O to form H_2CO_3 (Carbonic Acid) which is an acid. This makes CO_2 a reliable indicator of acidosis.*

   b. HCO_3 (Bicarb) is Basic, so more HCO_3 makes the ABG more Alkalotic (moves right)

2. If Acidotic (<7.35) look at the CO_2 levels.
   - If CO_2 levels are >45, it is a Respiratory Acidosis
   - If CO_2 levels are normal or <35, it is not a Respiratory Acidosis (it is likely a metabolic acidosis)

3. If Alkalotic (>7.45) look at the HCO_3levels.
   - If HCO_3 >26, it is a Metabolic Alkalosis
   - If HCO_3 is normal or <22, it is not a Metabolic Acidosis (it is a likely Respiratory Alkalosis)

4. Is it compensated?

   a. The compensatory mechanism is the opposite of the primary problem
      - An acidosis is compensated by HCO_3 (bicarb)
      - An alkalosis is compensated by CO_2 (acid)

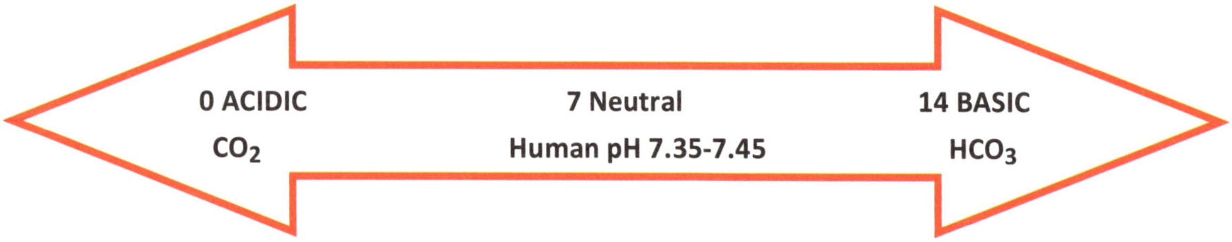

Acid-Base Disorder	Primary Change	Compensatory Response
Respiratory Acidosis <7.35	↑CO_2 >45	↑HCO_3 >26
Respiratory Alkalosis >7.45	↓CO_2 <35	↓HCO_3 <22
Metabolic Acidosis <7.35	↓HCO_3 <22	↓CO_2 <35
Metabolic Alkalosis >7.45	↑HCO_3 >26	↑CO_2 >45

Acid / Base Balance

Buffer Systems

- Bicarb (HCO_3)/ Carbonic Acid (H_2CO_3) — react in seconds
- Lungs blow off/hold CO_2 — react in minutes
- Kidneys resorb/excrete bicarb (HCO_3) — react in hours to days

CO2 Transport and Removal

CO_2 is a byproduct of metabolism

- Diffusion into circulation and transport to pulmonary capillaries
- Diffusion across capillary/alveolar membrane into the alveoli
- Cardiac Output moves the blood to the tissues
- Minute volume to blow off CO_2
    - CO_2 regulation is a function of MINUTE VOLUME (tidal volume [Vt] x respiratory rate [F])

Metabolic Alkalosis

pH > 7.35, Bicarb >26

Too little H+ or too much HCO_3

- Usually the result of H+, K+, NA+, CL- Loss
- Common causes are vomiting, Nasogastric (NG) suctioning, diuretics, corticosteroids, antacid poisoning, Diamox
- Treat the underlying cause

Metabolic Acidosis

pH <7.35 Bicarb <22

Too much H+ or too little HCO_3

- #1 cause is lactic acidosis (lactate >4)
- Ketoacidosis- diabetics/alcoholics
- Treat the underlying cause

Respiratory Alkalosis

pH > 7.45 CO_2 <35

- This is a result of alveolar hyperventilation (breathing too fast)
- Increased pH, decreased CO_2 (<35)
- Often caused by ASA poisoning (respiratory center stimulant), or Hyperthermia (heat injuries, hypermetabolic states, fever)
- If on a ventilator, check tidal volume first, then rate (Vt- volume, F- rate)

Respiratory Acidosis

pH < 7.35 CO_2 >45

- This is the result of a failure to remove CO_2 (breathing too slow)
- Causes include: chest wall injury, CNS depression, lung injury
- Decreased pH, Increased CO_2 (>45)

Anion Gap Acidosis

Sodium (+), Chloride (-), and Bicarb (-) are added together to determine the "Anion Gap"

- **Anion Gap** = (Na+) - (Cl- + HCO_3-)
- If ≥16 the patient has an anion gap metabolic acidosis
    - Normal Anion Gap is 12 (+/- 4)

The worse the gap (indicated by a larger number), the worse the acidosis

"Profound Anion Gap Acidosis" – Causes below

Underlying Cause	Offending Agent	Treatment
Methanol	(Alcohol poisoning)	IV Ethanol (ETOH) or Fomepizole
Uremia	(Kidney failure)	Dialysis
DKA	(Diabetic Ketoacidosis)	IV Fluid Resuscitation & Insulin
Propylene Glycol	(Liquid agent used in Diazepam/Lorazepam)	Flumazenil (Romazicon)
Isoniazid (INH)/**I**ron	(Tuberculosis medication/Iron supplements)	INH- Pyridoxine Iron-Deferoxamine
Lactate	(From anaerobic metabolism)	Correct inadequate tissue perfusion
Ethylene Glycol	(Antifreeze)	IV Ethanol (ETOH) or Fomepizole
Salicylates	(Aspirin)	Bicarb/Dialysis

Anion Gap Acidosis Treatment

- Ventilation must be secured before treatment (then **treat the underlying cause**)
- If the patient has a high anion gap acidosis with an unknown cause, treat with Narcan and Flumazenil
- Bicarb as a life sustaining rescue strategy if pH <7.0 (**treat the underlying cause first**)
    - Dosing based on severity of Acidosis

Basic Metabolic Panel

(Chem 7)

Na+ **135-145**mEq/L (Sodium)

Primary Extracellular Cation, helps nerves and muscles interact

K+ **3.5 – 5.0** mEq/L (Potassium)

Primary intracellular cation, responsible for cell excitability, resting membrane potential, etc. (MOST DANGEROUS ABNORMALITY)

Cl- **95-105** mEq/L (Chloride)

Extracellular anion, maintains osmotic pressure, helps stomach produce hydrochloric acid

CO_2 **22-26** mEq/L (Carbon Dioxide)

Important for helping maintain acid-base balance

BUN **6-24** mg/dL (Blood Urea Nitrogen)

Helps provide a picture of Renal {kidney} clearance

Cr **.7 to 1.4** mg/dL (Creatinine)

Helps provide a picture of Renal {kidney} clearance

Glucose 80-120 mg/dL (Blood sugar)

How much glucose (sugar) is circulating in the blood

Chem 7 Shorthand

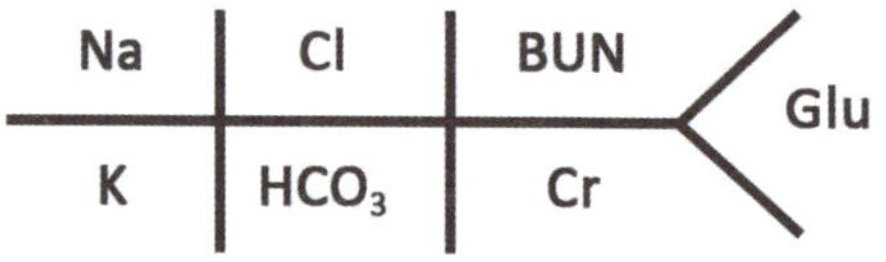

Chem 7 (BMP)	Normal Range
Na+	135 - 145
K+	3.5 - 5
Cl-	95 - 105
HCO_3	22 - 26
BUN	6 - 24
Cr	.7 - 1.4
Glucose	80 - 120

CBC
(Complete Blood Count)

HGB/HCT 15/45	(Hemoglobin/Hematocrit)
PLT 150k – 400k	(Platelets)
WBC 5k – 10k	(White Blood Cells)

- CBC-primary serum protein is albumin, produced by the liver (maintains colloid osmotic pressure)

CBC Shorthand

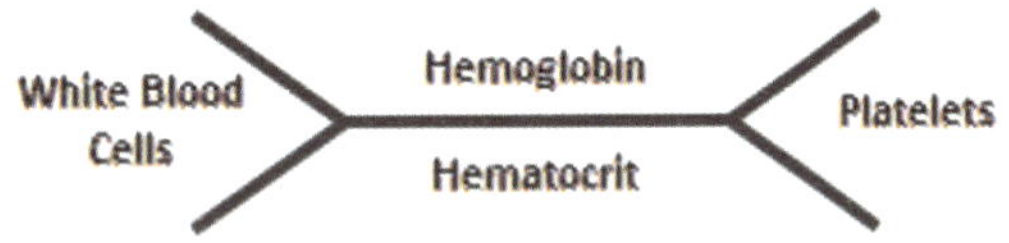

Coagulation
"Coag Panel"

PT 11 sec	(Prothrombin Time)	*extrinsic pathway*
PTT 21 - 35 sec	(Partial Thromboplastin Time)	*intrinsic pathway*
INR 1.0	(International Normalized Ratio)	

Heparin/Low Molecular Weight Heparin (Lovenox): Affects the intrinsic Pathway
Overdose treated with Protamine Sulfate

Coumadin (Warfarin): Affects the Extrinsic Pathway, clinically monitored by measuring INR.
Therapeutic INR typically 3-4
Overdose treated with Vitamin K

Memory tip: "You do PT outside to go to war and kill"
PT= Extrinsic pathway (doing PT outside)
War= Warfarin (Warfarin and Coumadin are the same thing)
Kill= The extrinsic pathway is Vitamin K dependent

Urine Output
"2/1/0.5"

Infant **2**cc/kg/hr

Child **1**cc/kg/hr

Adult **0.5** cc/kg/hr

- Average urine output for an adult is 30-50cc/hr
- Remember that cc (cubic centimeters) and mL (milliliters) are the same thing!

Osmolarity

- Osmolarity is the measure of solute concentration
  - Defined as the number of osmoles (Osm) of solute per liter (L) of solution
- Normal serum osmolality 280-295 mOsm/L
- Osmolality of blood increases with dehydration and decreases with over hydration
  - This is an EXTREMELY basic explanation

Medical Emergencies (16)

DKA

(**D**iabetic **K**eto**a**cidosis)

- Most common in Type I diabetic teens/children
- Elevated glucose (>350mg/dl)
- Elevated Ketones (ketosis) *this is what causes fruity breath*
- **ACIDOTIC** (metabolic acidosis)
- Kussmaul's respirations

Kussmaul's Respirations

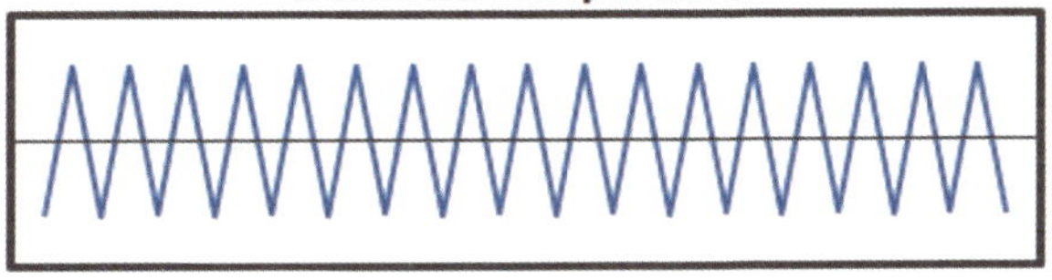

- First line treatment is fluid administration, then IV insulin to reduce blood glucose levels
- Average fluid deficit is 3-6L
- Administer Regular IV Insulin (Humilin or Novolin, both are short acting)
    - Do not lower glucose >100mg/dl per hour, do not lower less than 250mg/dL total
- Allowing blood glucose to drop to hypoglycemic levels is a common mistake that usually results in a rebound ketosis derived by counter-regulatory hormones
- Rapid correction of hyperglycemia and hyperosmolarity may shift water rapidly to the hyperosmolar intracellular space and may induce cerebral edema.

HHNK

(**H**yperglycemic **H**yperosmolar **N**on-**K**etosis)

- Common with Type II Diabetes
- Extremely elevated glucose (>600mg/dL) *sometimes >1000mg/dL*
- Normal ketones (non-ketotic)
- **NON-ACIDOTC**
- First line treatment is fluid administration, then IV insulin to reduce blood glucose levels
    - Average fluid deficit is 7-10L
- Administer Regular IV Insulin (Humilin or Novolin, both are short acting)
    - Do not lower glucose >100mg/dl per hour, do not lower less than 250mg/dL total
- Treat hypokalemia if present (60mg oral or 10mg IV potassium, oral route is preferred)

SIADH
(Syndrome of Inappropriate Anti-Diuretic Hormone)

- ADH = Anti-Diuretic Hormone (Desmopressin)
  - There is too much of this hormone in the body
- Hyponatremia is the problem (Na <135meq/L)
  - <130meq/L = Symptoms typically begin
  - <120 meq/L = Coma
- Tx with Hypertonic saline if symptomatic (do not exceed 0.5 meq/l/hr)
  - Can lead to central pontine myelinolysis (CPM) if Sodium is corrected too quickly
  - CPM is Irreversible brain damage evidenced by cerebral palsy, quadriplegia, death
- ORAL FLUID RESTRICTION (500 to 1,000 mL/day)
  - This is to prevent a dilutional hyponatremia

DI
(Diabetes Insipidus)

- A condition that occurs when the kidneys are unable to conserve water

Central DI: Not enough ADH is secreted by the pituitary gland
Nephrogenic DI: The kidneys do not respond to ADH

- Also caused by of Dilantin overdose and head injuries.

- **P**olydipsia (excessive thirst)
- **P**olyuria (excessive urination)
- **P**olyphagia (excessive hunger)

- 1st line treatment is IV fluid resuscitation (typically there is a 9L fluid deficit)
- Treat with Vasopressin / Desmopressin (DDAVP) to retain fluids

Esophageal Varicies

- Bleeding in the esophagus, most commonly due to chronic alcoholism (cirrhosis)
- Vomiting bright red blood (hematemesis)
    - Bright red diarrhea (hematochezia)
    - Patient often presents with syncope
    - Altered mental status due to hypovolemia
- **Life threatening!**
- Treat with Octreotide (Sandostatin)
    - Octreotide reduces splanchnic (spleen) and hepatic (liver) blood flow, and reduces variceal pressures
- Check Coagulation Values (PT/PTT/INR) to help anticipate the need for blood products
- Balloon Tamponade- a Sengstaken Blakemore tube can be placed to provide direct pressure on the bleeding (patient must be intubated first)
- DO NOT INSERT A NASOGASTRIC TUBE (can cause a lethal rupture of varicies)

Mallory Weiss/Boerhaave's Tears

- Rupture of the esophagus
- Commonly caused by chronic forceful vomiting (alcoholism, bulimia)
    - Presents with hematemesis
    - Often self-resolving (not life threatening)
    - If bleeding continues, treat like esophageal varicies
- Can cause mediastinitis secondary to leak of gastric contents into the chest
- Requires EGD (Esophagogastroduodenoscopy)
    - Gold standard

Hyperthyroidism/Grave's Dz / Thyrotoxicosis
("Thyroid Storm")

- Patient often presents with weight loss, palpitations, nervousness, *heat* intolerance
- Patient often has Exophthalmos (also called proptosis) which is a bulging of the eye
- Avoid ASA (Aspirin)
    - ASA prevents binding of thyroglobulin, making the situation worse
- Treatment:
    - Give IV fluids first!
    - Beta Blockers (Propanolol)
    - Steroids (Dexamethasone)
    - Tylenol for fever

Hypothyroidism/Myxedema Coma

- Patient presents with fatigue, *cold intolerance*, weight gain, puffy eyelids, sparse hair, possibly goiter
- Primarily occurs in women
- > 90% cases in winter (because the patient has cold intolerance and is now suffering from hypothermia)
- Officially "Myxedema Coma" upon LOC change
- Tx with IV Levothyroxine (T4) or Triostat (T3)
    - Levothyroxine is "Synthroid"

Cushing's Syndrome

- Buffalo hump, moon face, thin arms and legs, purple striae on abdomen
- Causes:
    - Excessive use of corticosteroids (iatrogenic- condition caused by treatment)
    - Tumor
- Usually resolves when corticosteroids are stopped or tumor is removed

Adrenal Insufficiency /Adrenal Crisis

(Addison's Dz)

- Patient often presents with depression, malaise, *salt craving*
- Patient will often have bronze colored skin *(JFK had Addison's)*
- Treated with oral steroids (Prednisone)
- Negative Adrenocorticotropic hormone (ACTH) testing, also known as corticotropin or cosyntropin test
- No Etomidate in RSI (due to adrenal suppression)

Liver Failure

- Caused by hepatitis, alcoholism, Tylenol overdose, etc.
- INR > 1.5 (due to decreased Albumin and coagulation factor production)
- Liver breaks down ammonia
- Increased ammonia leads to increased ICP
- Treatment is mainly supportive
- Treat with Lactulose (removes ammonia)

Hepatic Encephalopathy

- Any disease process affecting normal liver functions can lead to hepatic encephalopathy
- Various neurologic symptoms including changes in consciousness, behavior changes, and personality changes

Asterixis :

- Coarse "flapping" muscle tremor may be observed during voluntary movement
- This is from the loss of fine motor skills often seen with Hepatic Encephalopathy
- Treat with Lactulose

Septic Shock

- Someone who is in shock 2° to sepsis (infection in the bloodstream)
- Hypotensive with *normal heart rate*
- Hypotensive while being refractory to fluids
- Patient needs IV fluid therapy and vasopressors
- Levophed (Norepinephrine) is vasopressor of choice in profound hypotension
- Do not use Etomidate in RSI (due to its adrenal suppression)

Pancreatitis

- Pain that is usually centered in the upper middle or upper left abdomen. Often radiates from the front of the abdomen through to the back, begins or worsens after eating, lasts a few days, and may feel worse when a person lies flat on his or her back.
- The digestive enzymes in the pancreas are destroying the pancreas
- Increased lipase levels (usually >3 times normal)

Grey-Turner's Sign: Flank ecchymosis caused by hemorrhagic pancreatitis

Cullen's Sign: Periumbilical ecchymosis caused by hemorrhagic pancreatitis

- Demerol for pain (because Morphine can cause spasms of the Sphincter of Oddi)
- Typically requires surgery

Hyperkalemia

(K+ >5.0)

- Caused by either increased intake or decreased excretion of Potassium
- Patient may present with abdominal cramps, nausea, hypotension, bradycardia, numbness (especially in the legs
- EKG will show "Tall," "Tented," or "Peaked" T-Waves
- Treatment
    - Push K+ into the cells with Bicarb, Insulin, D50, Albuterol
    - Excrete excess K+ with Lasix and Kayexalate through urine (lasix), and feces (kayexalate)
    - Prevent V-Tach with Calcium Gluconate

- K+ will change about 0.6meq for every 0.1 change in pH

Hyperkalemia = Tall, Tented, Peaked T waves

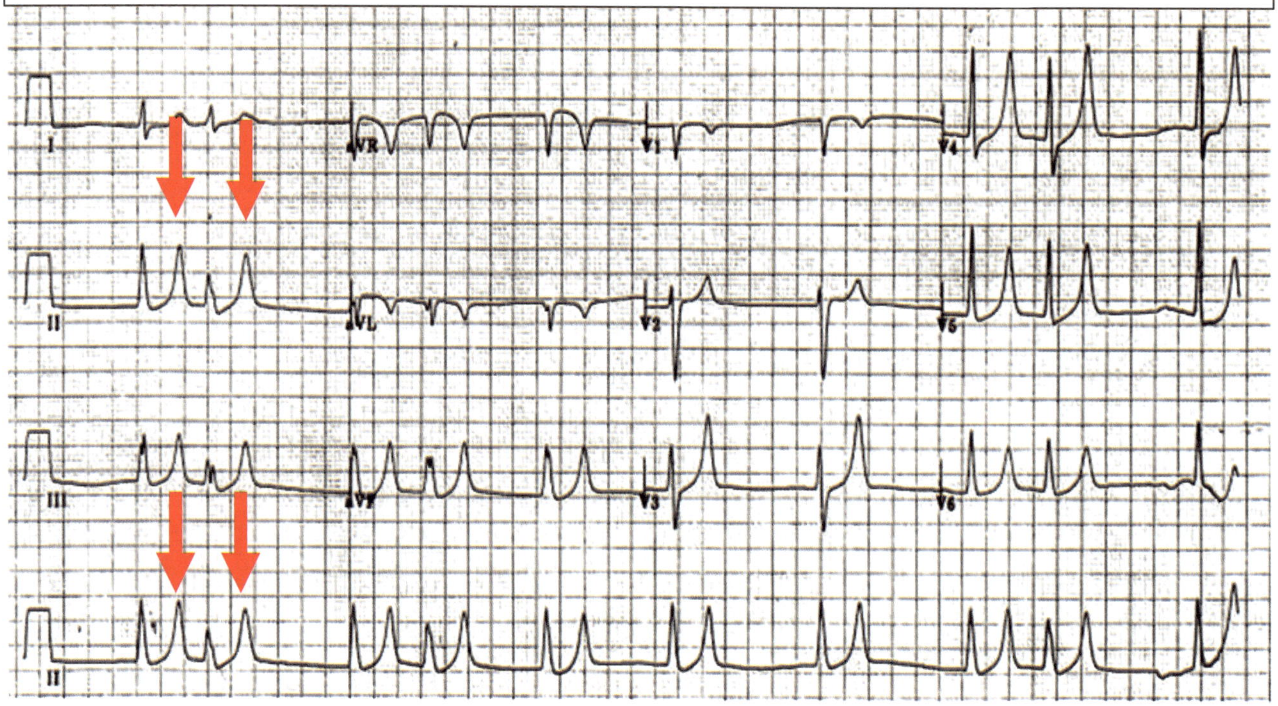

Hypokalemia

K+ <3.5

- Pt. often presents with malaise, weakness, history of poor dietary intake
- Lasix is a common iatrogenic cause of hypokalemia
- EKG will show "Depressed," "Inverted," of "Flattened" T Waves
- Give oral potassium 60 mEq (preferred route)
- If hypokalemia is severe, can give 10mEq IV potassium
    - NEVER give as a bolus (could be fatal)
    - IV Potassium is what is used in lethal injections

Hypokalemia = Depressed, Inverted, or Flattened T waves

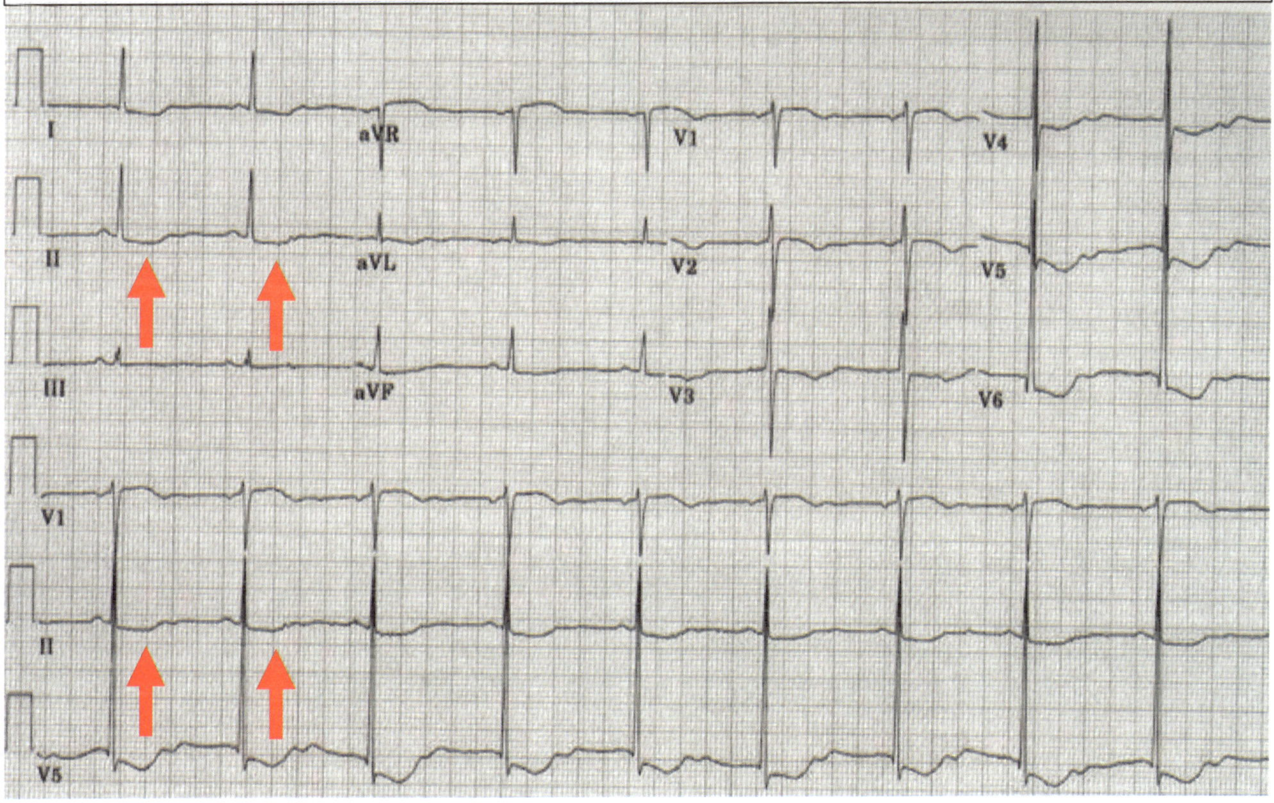

Hypocalcemia

Ca <8.2mg/dL

- Decreased Calcium or Vitamin D intake/ increased calcium excretion/Hyperparathyroidism
- Anxiety, confusion, delirium
- Hyperactive Deep Tendon Reflexes (DTRs 3+ or 4+)
- Prolonged QT interval on EKG, narrow QRS, possible U wave

Chvosteks Sign: cheek muscle spasms when the facial nerve (CN VII) tapped

Trousseue's Sign: forearm tetany when B/P cuff is applied

- Treat with Calcium Gluconate
    - Do not bolus, can lead to hypotension, syncope, arrhythmias

Peripheral Vascular Disease (PVD)

Deep Venous Thrombosis (DVT)

Virchow's Triad Δ Virchow=Venous

- Loss of vein integrity (surgery, trauma)
- Stasis (long seated ride, hospital bed)
- Hypercoagulable state (cancer, pregnancy)

- Aching pain, **WARM**, red, and swollen
  - Blood is getting into the limb, it just can't get out. This is why the limb is warm

Homan's Sign – dorsiflexion of the foot and constriction of the calf causing calf pain

- Treatment: Lovenox or Coumadin

Arterial Occlusion

- Usually embolic (from DVT or clot in the heart)
- Presents with claudication (latin for "limping"). This is cramping pain felt in the extremities, usually referenced in how many blocks someone walks before the pain occurs (i.e. pain after walking a single block would be "1 Block Claudication")
- COLD Limb
  - Blood is not getting into the limb, this is why it is cold

6 P's of Arterial Occlusion

Pain	Early finding
Pallor	"Pale skin"
Paresthesia	Numbness
Poikilothermia	"Cold blooded"
Pulselessness	Late finding
Paralysis	Late finding

Poikilothermia: body temperature that varies with its surroundings

- Treatment
  - Non-Surgical: Smoking cessation, lipid control, exercise
  - Surgical: Only if life or limb-threatening condition exists

Environmental Injuries (4) /Toxicology (6)

Crotalinae (Pit Viper) Snakes

- Rattlesnakes, Copperheads, Water Moccasins
- Localized fang marks, pain, swelling, tachycardia, tachypnea, oral numbness, coagulopathy
- DO NOT use tourniquets
- Give antivenom (CroFab, FabAV), can often require 4-6 vials per patient

Patients with Thermoregulatory Problems

- Pediatric
- Paralyzed
- Head Injuries
  - Diffuse Axonal Injury (Coma)
- Burn victims

Hypothermia

(Cold Injuries)

- Defined as a core temp below 35° C (95° F)
- Paradoxical undressing is a hallmark sign of hypothermia (due to delirium)
- Shivering is limited by glycogen stores (stops at core temp of 32° C / 89.6° F)
- Treat with passive external and active external rewarming first!
- Heated blankets, HPMK, etc.
- If unsuccessful, treat with active internal rewarming
- Heated IV fluids, warming packs, GI lavage with warmed fluids, etc.
- IV fluids should be warmed to 39° C (102.2° F)

After Drop: return of cold blood to the core induced by external rewarming and peripheral vasodilation

- Dysrhythmia in hypothermia- caused by an increase in lactate and K+ levels
  - Cardiac irritability begins at 33° C (91.4° F)
  - "Osborn Wave", "J Wave," or "Hypothermia Hump" on EKG

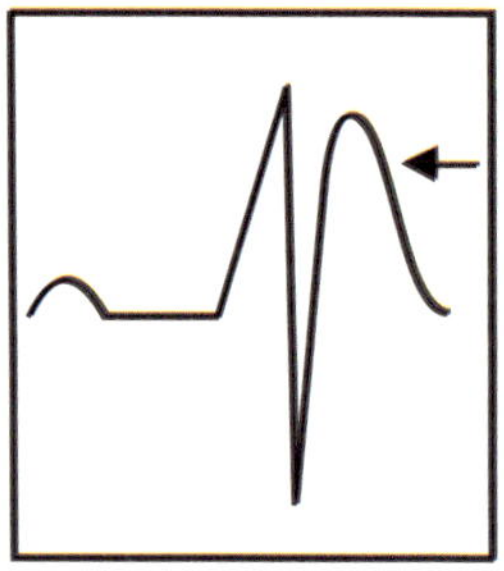

Hyperthermia
(Heat Injuries)

- Heat Cramps, Heat Exhaustion, and Heat Stroke
- Heat cramps caused by Hyponatremia
    - Primary cation lost in heat injuries is Sodium (Na+)
- Heat exhaustion typically occurs at core temps > 40° C (104° F)
    - Patient often has respiratory alkalosis due to hyperventilation (blowing off CO_2)
    - With heat exhaustion there is no neurologic impairment
- Heat stroke is *any* heat injury with LOC change (patient doesn't have to stop sweating to be a heat stroke)
- Administer crystalloid fluids (NS/LR)for volume replacement (minimum 2 liters)
    - Never use colloids for heat injuries (Hextend/Hespan)

Dehydration

Blood
- ↑Hematocrit (HCT)
- ↑Blood Urea Nitrogen (BUN)

Urine
- ↑ Specific Gravity (SG)
- Ketones (Ketonuria)

"The blood and the urine are more concentrated due to fluid loss"
- Give a minimum of 2L crystalloids (LR/NS)

Drowning

- Hypothermia is a concern in warm and cold water drowning

Cold Water
- Dry drowning (due to laryngospasms)
- Spinal immobilization

Mammalian diving reflex: apnea, bradycardia, and vasoconstriction to maintain cerebral perfusion that occurs in cold water drowning (mainly in children)

Warm Water
- Wet drowning
- Spinal immobilization

High Altitude Injuries

Acute Mountain Sickness (AMS): typically occurs in those that are not acclimatized and have recently traveled to altitude (within 24 hours). Symptoms have been reported as low as 6,900ft MSL (but usually occurs above 8,000ft MSL), and often resolves within a few days of ascent.

- Not life threatening
- Symptoms: headache, nausea, vomiting, lassitude (feeling weak)
- Treatment: if possible, descend at least 1,000ft to 3,000ft (<8,000ft MSL optimal), hydration, Acetazolamide (Diamox), Tylenol/Motrin for headache, Phenergan/Zofran for nausea, Dexamethasone (Decadron, 4-8mg IM) if symptoms persist

High Altitude Pulmonary Edema (HAPE): onset occurs 2-4 days after rapid ascent > 10,000 ft.

- Symptoms: rales, tachycardia, tachypnea, dyspnea at rest, non-productive cough (although can have pink frothy sputum)
- Potentially life threatening
- Treatment: descend, Acetazolamide (Diamox), Dexamethasone (Decadron), Nifedipine (promotes pulmonary vasculature dilation), Oxygen, Hyperbaric therapy (Gamow Bag)

High Altitude Cerebral Edema (HACE): often concurrent with AMS or HAPE (although this is not required), often at altitudes >12,000 ft. MSL in climbers who ascend rapidly. Occurs the latest of all altitude injuries, typically after 5 days at sustained high altitudes.

- LIFE THREATENING
- Symptoms: visual changes, parasthesias (numbness), mental status changes, coma
- Treatment: descend, Acetazolamide (Diamox), Dexamethasone (Decadron), Oxygen, Hyperbaric therapy (Gamow Bag)

Rhabdomyolysis

"Rhabdo"

- Can be caused by crush injuries, hyperthermia, excessive exercise, drugs, etc.
- The breakdown of muscle fibers that leads to the release of muscle fiber contents (myoglobin) into the bloodstream
- Myoglobin is harmful to the kidneys
  - Patient usually has dark cola or tea colored urine (myoglobinuria)
- Creatinine Kinase (CK) will be greatly elevated (≥ 5 times normal levels)
- First line treatment is crystalloid IV fluid resuscitation
  - Bicarb (Alkalinizes the urine, prevents cast formation in the kidneys)
  - Lasix (Loop diuretic)
  - Mannitol (Osmotic diuretic)

Overdoses & Toxidromes

Acetylsalicylic Acid "ASA" Poisoning

(Aspirin)

- Nausea, vomiting, *ringing in the ears (Tinnitus)*
- ASA poisoning can cause respiratory alkalosis (it is a respiratory center stimulant)
- Respiratory alkalosis progresses to metabolic acidosis (mixed disturbance)
- Can lead to Reye's syndrome in peds (potentially fatal liver and brain damage)
    - Liver fails causing ↑ammonia levels, which ↑ICP and leads to encephalopathy
- Treat with Bicarb (to correct acidosis)
    - Dialysis can be helpful

Tylenol Poisoning

(Each stage lasts 24hrs)

- Stage I – Flu symptoms
- Stage II – Flu sx stop, liver failure occurs, RUQ pain, increased liver enzymes
- Stage III – Peak liver enzymes, RUQ pain, Flu symptoms (DEATH STAGE)
- Stage IV – Resolution period
    - Treat with Mucomyst *N*-acetylcysteine, abbreviated "NAC"
    - Trade name Acetadote "acetaminophen antidote"

Dilantin Overdose

- Dilantin (Phenytoin) is used to treat and prevent seizures
- Overdose can cause Supraventricular Tachycardia (SVT) and Ventricular dysrhythmias
- Coma, confusion, tremors
- Dilantin overdose can cause Diabetes Insipidus (DI) like symptoms
    - treat under Diabetes Insipidus protocols
- Supportive care (airway, IV, O2)
- Gastric Lavage (charcoal use is controversial)

Iron Overdose

- Typically from elemental iron supplements
- Common in children
- Antidote is Deferoxamine
    - Pink urine "*vin rose urine*" indicates a therapeutic level of Deferoxamine

Beta Blocker Overdose

Drugs like: Labetolol, Carvidolol, and Esmolol

- Symptoms- hypotension, bradycardia, conduction delays
- Glucagon is the antidote
- Consider cardiac pacing
    - Fluids for hypotension

Calcium Channel Blocker Overdose

Drugs like: Amlodipine, Verapamil, Cardizem, and Diltiazem

- Symptoms- Hypotension, bradycardia, conduction delays
- Calcium Gluconate is the antidote
    - Fluids for hypotension

Digitalis Toxicity

- Flu like symptoms, visual disturbances
    - Yellow / Green halos (life looks like Van Gogh paintings)
- Slurred upslope on QRS
- Treat with Digibind (Digoxin Immune Fab)
    - Avoid electricity (cardioversion, pacing, etc.)

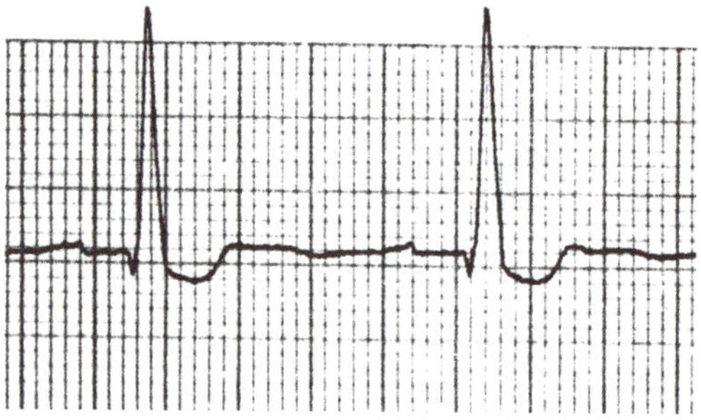

Tricyclic Antidepressant (TCA) overdose

Drugs like: Amitriptyline (Elavil) Nortriptyline (Pamelor)

- Patients with a TCA overdose often present with an anticholinergic-like toxidrome
- Tachycardia and widened QRS common, prolonged QT intervals
    - Torsades de Pointes occurs after prolonged QT interval
- Treatment is Bicarb
    - Dialysis is not helpful
    - DO NOT use Physostigmine

TCA Overdose = Prolonged QT Intervals
(normal QT is < ½ of the R to R interval)

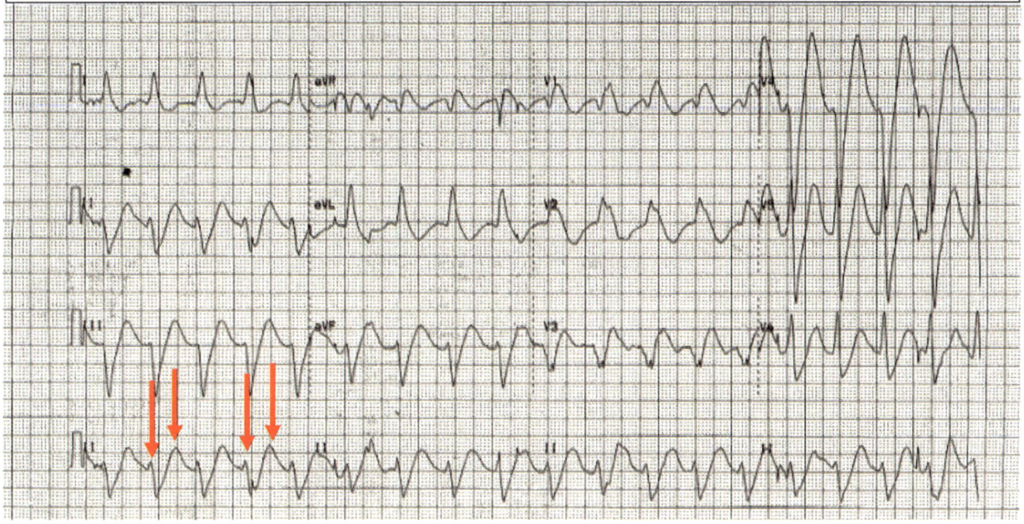

Alcohol Poisoning

- Drinking too much alcohol (liquor, wine, beer)
- Hypoglycemia is common in alcoholics (due to poor dietary intake)
- Treatment is supportive (protect the airway, IV fluids, etc.)
- If seizures occur from withdrawals (Delirium Tremens) give Valium

Ethylene Glycol / Methanol Poisoning

- Ethylene Glycol- antifreeze
- Methanol - methyl alcohol, wood alcohol, sterno (canned fuel)
- Causes profound anion-gap acidosis (≥16)
- Treat with IV ethanol (ETOH)
  - Competes with methanol to avoid conversion to toxic metabolites (formic acid)
  - Metabolites cause central nervous system poisoning
- Treat with Fomepizole (Antizol)
  - DO NOT use Fomepizole if IV ETOH has been infused (it prolongs the ETOH half-life)

Hydrocarbons

- Drinking volatile chemicals like gasoline, diesel, paint stripper, etc.
- Decreased viscosity leads to aspiration
- Aspiration causes chemical pneumonitis
- Intubate
- DO NOT induce vomiting

Organophosphate Toxicity

"Cholinergic Poisoning"

- Common in those who work with pesticides, farmers
- Causes the inhibition of acetylcholinesterase (AChE), leading to the accumulation of acetylcholine (ACh) in the body
- Think of CBRNE (chemical agent poisoning)

SLUDGE

  - **S**alivation, **L**acrimation, **U**rination, **D**efecation, **G**astrointestinal, **E**mesis

- Treatment
  - Atropine (anticholinergic)
  - 2-Pam Chloride "2-Pam Crowbar," pulls the organophosphate off the ACh
  - If seizures are present, use a Benzo (Valium/Ativan/Versed)

Anticholinergic Poisoning

Drugs like: Atropine, scopolamine (motion sickness), Chlorpheniramine (Deconamine), Hydroxyzine (Atarax), Dimenhydrinate (Dramamine), Diphenhydramine (Benadryl), Meclizine (Antivert), Promethazine (Phenrgan)

- Physostigmine is the antidote
- Initial: 0.5-2 mg slow IVP (not to exceed 1 mg/min); keep atropine nearby for immediate use
- If no response, repeat q20min PRN

Cyanide Toxicity

- Causes a coma with seizures, apnea, and cardiac arrest, with death following in a matter of minutes.
- Common in Jewelers (they use it to clean jewelry)
- United States standard cyanide antidote kit first uses a small inhaled dose of amyl nitrite, followed by intravenous sodium nitrite, followed by intravenous sodium thiosulfate
- Hydroxocobalamin is newly approved in the US and is available in Cyanokit antidote kits (www.cyanokit.com)

Cocaine Overdose

- Tachycardia, elevated temps, miosis (constricted pupils), hyperthermia
- Antidote is benzos- Valium, Ativan, Verse
- Do not give β blockers (leads to unopposed α adrenergic activity)
  - DO NOT use drugs like Esmolol, Propanolol, etc.

Benzodiazepine Overdose

Drugs like: Valium, Ativan, Versed

- Use Romazicon (Flumazenil)
  - Pushing Romazicon too fast can lead to seizures!
- Remember the ½ life of the benzo is usually longer than the ½ life of the Romazicon (½ life approx. 40 to 80 minutes)

Opioid Overdose

Drugs like: MS Contin, Oxycodone, Norco, Fentanyl, Morphine, Demerol, Percocet, etc.

- Use Naloxone (Narcan)
- Any altered mental status, consider use of Narcan
- Remember the ½ life of the opioid is usually longer than the ½ life of Narcan
    - Narcan ½ life is approximately 45 minutes
- When pushing Narcan , use the lowest dose possible to avoid complete blockade of the opioid receptors

Toxic Agent	Treatment/Antidote
Alkalis	Copious Water
Anticholinergics	Physostigmine
ASA	Bicarb
Benzodiazepines	Flumazenil (Romazicon)
Beta Blockers	Glucagon
Calcium Channel Blockers	Calcium Gluconate
Carbon Monoxide (CO)	Oxygen & Hyperbaric Chamber
Cocaine	Benzodiazepines
Coumadin (Warfarin)	Vitamin K
Crotalinae (Pit Viper)	CroFab, FabAV
Cyanide	Sodium Thiosulfate/Sodium Nitrite/ Amyl Nitrate
Digitalis	Digibind/ Digoxin Immune Fab
Dilantin	Supportive Care
Ethylene Glycol	IV Ethanol or Fomezipole
Heparin/LMWH (Lovenox)	Protamine Sulfate
Hydrocarbons	Intubate
Hydroflouric Acid	Calcium Gluconate
Isoniazid (INH)	Pyridoxine
Iron	Deferoxamine
Methanol	IV Ethanol or Fomezipole
Opiods	Naloxone (Narcan)
Organophosphates	Atropine & 2-Pam Chloride
Tricyclic Antidepressants (TCAs)	Bicarb
Tylenol	Mucomyst/Acetadote

Burns (5)

1st Degree	(sunburns)
2nd Degree "partial thickness"	(blisters)
3rd Degree "full thickness"	(completely destroyed tissue)

Burn Formulas

Brooke 2ccx kg x BSA = fluids over 24hrs (1st half in 1st 8 hours from time of burn)

Universal 2-4ccx kg x BSA = fluids over 24hrs (1st half in 1st 8 hours from time of burn)
Also called the "Consensus Formula"

Parkland 4cc x kg x BSA = fluids over 24hrs (1st half in 1st 8 hours from time of burn)

Only count 2nd and 3rd degree burns
Parkland is the preferred formula
Lactated Ringers is the preferred fluid

Child body Part	% of total BSA
Arm	9%
Head and neck	18%
Leg	14%
Anterior trunk	18%
Posterior trunk	18%

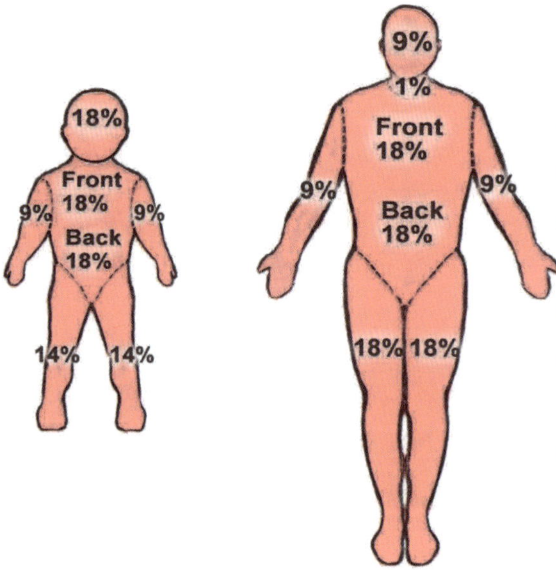

Adult body Part	% of total BSA
Arm	9%
Head	9%
Neck	1%
Leg	18%
Anterior trunk	18%
Posterior trunk	18%

- The face is 4 ½ % BSA in the adult
- "Palmer Method" - The palm represents 1% BSA in both adults and children
- Average urine output for an adult is 30-50ml/hr
- Patients with burns >20% BSA can also have an adynamic ileus (decreased bowel movement)
    - This can cause problems in-flight due to the expansion of wet gasses is restricted (Boyle's Law)

Electrical Injuries

Predictors of severity= Voltage and Amperage (amperage is a better predictor)

- Low voltage <1000 volts
- High voltage >1000 volts

- Resistance of internal body structure and tissue (dense parts of the body resist injury better)
- Type of pathway and current
- Duration and intensity of contact
    - Most likely cause of death in electrical injuries is cardiac insult
    - Flexor crease burns are the hallmark of true conductive injury
    - Oral commissure (corners of the mouth) burns common in children <2 y/o
        - From biting electrical cords

Alternating Current (A/C)

- Household current in the US (110v A/C)
- Will cause continual muscle contractions
- Victim will be UNABLE TO PULL THEMSELVES AWAY!
- Explosive exit wound
- Causes V-Fib

Direct Current (D/C)

- Victim is able to pull themselves away from the current
- Discrete exit wound
- Causes asystole

Myoglobinuria is common in severe electrical injuries

- Treatment is similar to that of crush injuries
- Maintain a urine output of 100ml/h in order to perfuse the kidneys and prevent renal failure (acute tubular necrosis or ATN)
- Sodium Bicarb to correct acidosis (also increases solubility of myoglobin in urine)
- Mannitol to increase UOP and minimize ATN

Chemical Burns

- Any chemical burn patient should be flushed with copious water prior to transport if the patient is stable (irrigation takes priority over transport)

Acids

- Cause coagulative necrosis
- Dilute with copious amounts of water
- Neutralize hydrofluoric acid with calcium gluconate

Alkalis "Alkali = Liquefy"

- Dehydrate cells causing saponification (liquefaction necrosis)
- Dilute with copious amounts of water
- WORSE THAN ACID BURNS

Inhalational Burns

Supraglottic Injury results from *thermal* insult

- "Above the vocal cords"
- Facial burns, carbonaceous sputum, singed facial hair, stridor
- Treat with high flow 02, corticosteroids, supportive care

Infraglottic Injury results from *chemical* insult

- "Below the vocal cords"
- Increased pulmonary capillary permeability (leads to pulmonary edema)
  - High index of suspicion in any patient that is hypoxic despite O2 therapy
- Treat with high flow 02, corticosteroids, supportive care
  - Hyperbaric chamber if available

Carbon Monoxide (CO) intoxication

- Causes asphyxiation
- "Cherry Red Skin" due to carboxyhemoglobin
  - Histotoxic hypoxia
- Headache is a common finding (symptoms are based on degree of poisoning)
- Accounts for as much as 80% of fatalities from inhalation injury
  - Assume CO exposure if the patient was in an enclosed area
  - CO causes false high SPO2 readings (get an ABG)
- Any patient with CO poisoning needs 100% 02 (usually for 12-24 hours)

Synthetic Material Fires

- Fires involving the combustion of cellulose, nylon, wool, silk, asphalt, and polyurethane increase the risk for hydrogen cyanide poisoning
    - Histotoxic hypoxia
- Cyanide is released during the incomplete combustion of products such as plastics and acrylics (kids toys, carpet, office furniture)
    - Cyanide poisoning is treated with Sodium Thiosulfate and Amyl Nitrate and Sodium Nitrite
        - Alternative- Newly FDA approved Cyanokit (www.cyanokit.com)

Trauma (9)

Newton's 1st Law of Motion: Unless it is acted on by a force, a body at rest will remain at rest and a body in motion will move at constant speed in a straight line

Law of Inertia

Newton's 2nd Law of Motion: When a force is applied to a body, the body accelerates, and the acceleration is directly proportional to the force applied and inversely proportional to the mass of the body

Force = mass x acceleration

Newton's 3rd Law of Motion: For every action there is an equal and opposite reaction

Killers in Flight

- Tension Pneumothorax
- Pericardial Tamponade
- Hypovolemia

Gunshot Wounds

- High velocity weapons fire projectiles >2000 fps (feet per second)
    - Rifles
- Velocity is the most important factor in GSW damage

Weapon	Level	Velocity
Crossbow	Low	300 fps
Handgun	Moderate	900-1500 fps
Rifle	High	>2000 fps

Miscellaneous

- The most commonly damaged organ is the skin
- THE MOST DEFINTIVE ASSESSMENT OF SHOCK IS LACTIC ACIDOSIS (lactate >4)

Injury Patterns

Motor Vehicle Crash (MVC)

Side Impact

- Rib fractures,
    - Splenic rupture secondary to rib fracture (Hypovolemia, (+) Kehr's Sign)
- Clavicular fractures
- Femur fractures

Front Impact

- Rib fractures (with possible hemo/pneumothorax)
- Concussion, skull fracture
- Dislocated hips, acetabular fractures

Rear Impact

- T12-L1 most common back injury
    - T12 Fracture is also called a "Chance fracture," has increased chance of splenic injury
- C2 (Hangman's) Fracture also common

Rollover

- Unpredictable injury pattern
- Possible C1 (Jefferson's) Fracture from axial loading

- Lap belt injuries are evidenced by ecchymosis over the abdomen and chest
    - "Clasp knife effect"
- ANY seat belt bruising should cause a high index of suspicion for internal injury!

Motorcycle Crash

Front Impact

- All lower extremities from impact with handlebars while moving forward, abdominal injuries

Side Impact

- Open lower extremities fracture

"Other" Crashes

- ATVs: Clavicular and sternal Fx
- Snowmobiles: C2 (Hangman's) Fx

Falls

- Falls from 15-20 feet (or 3 x standing height) are associated with severe injury
- One Story home = 15 ft.
- Two Story home = 30 ft.
- Adults land on their feet if fall is >15 ft. (land on their head at <15 ft.)
- Calcaneal fractures
- Compression Fractures T10, T12-L1
- Bilateral wrist fractures (FOOSH- Fall on out-stretched hand)
    - FOOSH often causes a Colle's Fracture (distal radius)
- Children land on their head no matter what height
- This is due to their large heads

Abdominal Trauma

- Spleen Fracture/Rupture
    - Most commonly injured solid organ in blunt trauma
    - Most blunt trauma in the abdomen is due to MVC
    - Massive hemorrhage due to vascular supply of spleen

Kehr's Sign: Left shoulder irritation secondary to diaphragmatic irritation from blood

Balance Sign: Dullness to percussion on the left side of the abdomen due to coagulated blood

- Colon / Small intestine- Most commonly injured hollow organ from penetrating trauma
- Liver - Most commonly injured solid organ in penetrating trauma (stab wounds, GSW, shank)

Coopernails Sign: Scrotal or labial ecchymosis from abdominal trauma or pelvic fractures

Halstead's Sign: Marbled skin on the abdomen following abdominal trauma (caused by blood in the abdomen)

Diaphragmatic Hernia

- Most common cause is blunt force trauma during MVC
- Most commonly occurs on the left side (right side is protected partially by the liver)
- Abdominal contents are forced into the chest
- Bowels sounds auscultated during chest exam
- Scaphoid abdomen (looks like an empty bowl)

Genitourinary Trauma

- Involves the kidneys bladder, urethra and genitals
  - Usually from blunt force trauma
  - Suspect if patient has blood at the urethral meatus, blood in the scrotum (Coopernails sign), pelvic fracture, high riding or non-palpable prostate
  - Hematuria is the hallmark sign
- Blunt trauma to the bladder is highly associated with pelvic fractures
  - Lateral pelvic fracture (from MVC) rarely has life threatening bleeding
  - Unstable pelvic fracture is always life threatening! ("Open Book" with A/P force)
  - Vertical shear is the worst (due to the rupture of the great vessels)
- Blood at the urethral meatus is the most important sign of urethral injury
  - Urinary catheter is contraindicated

Chest Trauma

Cardiac Tamponade

- Accumulated fluid around the heart either due to blunt or penetrating trauma
  - >150mL of blood accumulation can be fatal

Kussmauls Sign- Rise in venous pressure on inspiration

Early Tamponade: Pulsus Paradoxis (drop in B/P 10-15mmHg on inspiration), tachycardia

- Treat with IV Fluids (to improve preload)

Late Tamponade: Beck's Triad presentation

- Treat with pericardiocentesis

Beck's Triad Δ

- Muffled heart tones
- Hypovolemia with narrowed pulse pressure (systolic and diastolic numbers are close together, ex 90/70)
- Jugular venous distention (JVD)

"Electrical Alternans" on EKG

- Remember, the EKG is a "camera." In electrical alternans the heart is getting closer to and further away from the camera as it moves around inside the sac of fluid (pericardium)

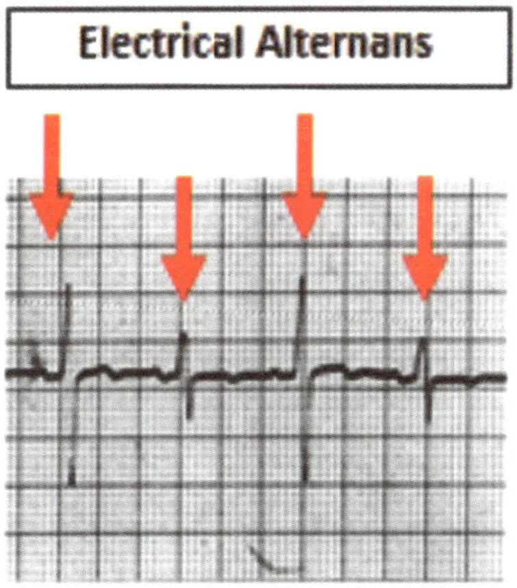

Pneumothorax

- Accumulation of air in the thoracic cavity, can be from blunt or penetrating trauma
    - Spontaneous pneumo is from rupture of blebs (tall, thin males)
    - Sudden increase in PPLAT indicates probable tension pneumo
    - Jugular Venous Distention (JVD) is a late sign (due to increased intrapleural pressures)
- In order to be a "Sucking Chest Wound" the chest wall defect must be >2/3 of the diameter of the trachea (air prefers to go into the hole in the chest as opposed to the trachea)

Initial Treatment: Occlusive dressing over the wound (Three sided)

- Needle decompression if symptomatic
    - $2^{nd}/3^{rd}$ ICS Mid-Clavicular Line (MCL)
    - 5th ICS Mid-Axillary Line (MAL)
    - Always guide the needle over the top of rib (avoids neurovascular bundle)

Definitive Treatment: Tube Thoracostomy (chest tube)

- 5th or 6th ICS Anterior Axillary Line (AAL)
    - Can use the Mid-Axillary Line (MAL) if the AAL is not an option

- 4th ICS AAL/MAL can lead to lung damage (too high)
- 7th ICS AAL/MAL can lead to splenic damage (too low)

Air accumulation in the chest
(air is black, fluids are white)

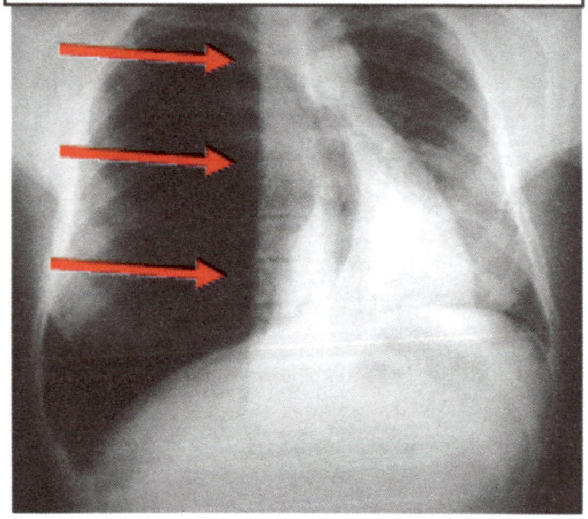

Hemothorax

- Accumulation of blood in the thoracic cavity
    - Often from a laceration of the Inferior Mammary Artery (IMA)
    - Massive Hemothorax is defined as >1500mL of blood (or 1/3 of patient's blood volume)

Treatment: Tube Thoracostomy (chest tube)

- 5^{th}or 6th ICS Anterior Axillary Line (AAL)
    - Can use the Mid-Axillary Line (MAL) if the AAL is not an option
- 4th ICS MAL can lead to lung damage (too high)
- 7th ICS MAL can lead to splenic damage (too low)

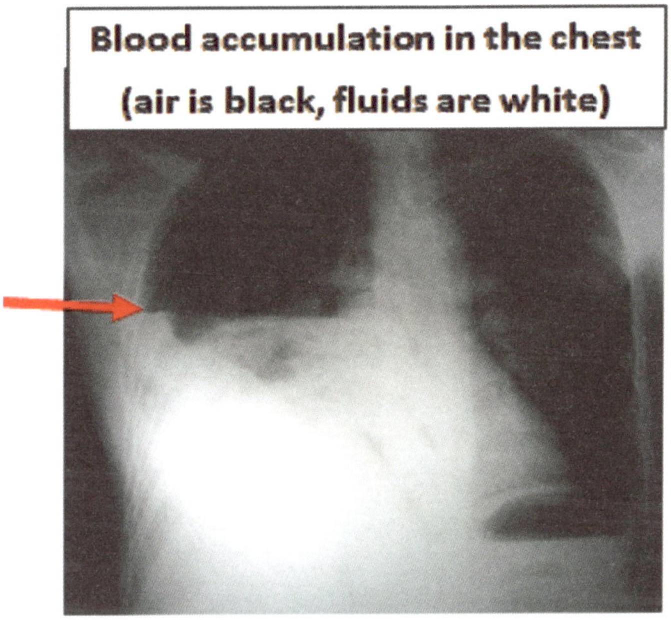

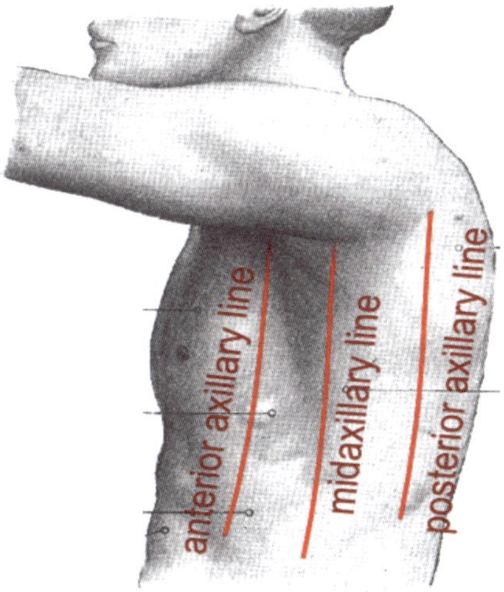

Rib Fracture

- Can be diagnosed clinically based on history and presentation
- Difficulty taking deep breaths is common
- $1^{st}/2^{nd}/3^{rd}$ Rib Fx associated with head, neck, spinal cord injuries
- $10^{th}/11^{th}/12^{th}$ Rib Fx associated with liver and spleen injuries
- Treat with analgesics and ensure the patient takes deep breaths (despite pain) to prevent atelectasis (lung tissue collapse)

Flail Chest

- Defined as 2 or more ribs broken in 2 or more places
- Associated with pulmonary contusion and paradoxical movement of flail segment
- Flail segment should be stabilized with tape and bulky dressings
    - Or place a sandbag on the chest (rarely done)
- High flow O_2
- Transport injured side down

Facial Trauma

- Avulsed teeth?- put in gauze soaked in NS, milk, or between the cheek and gum
- Tripod fracture- involves the Zygoma, most commonly at the zygomatic arch
- Hyphema- blood in the anterior chamber of the eye
- Tracheobronchial injury- presents with hoarseness, stridor, Hamman's Crunch

Hamman's Crunch- Crunching, rasping sound, synchronous with the heartbeat

Leforte Fractures

WATCH FOR AIRWAY COMPROMISE!

Le Forte I: Horizontal across the maxilla, maxilla and maxillary teeth are moveable

Le Forte II: Bridge of nose and around the mouth, usually from a downward blow to the nose

LeForte III: Transverse Fracture, aka "Craniofacial Disassociation" (goes through the orbits)

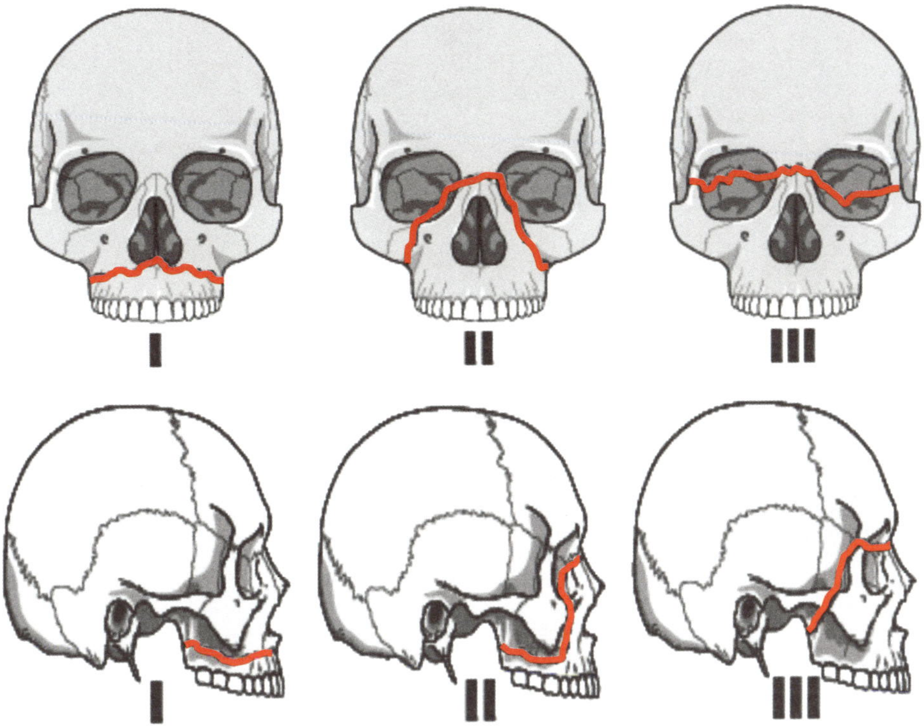

Fluid Resuscitation

- Fluids are used to bring up B/P in trauma (not vasopressors)
- Hypotension starts at 30% blood loss
- Average circulating blood volume in an adult is 5L (75ml/kg)

Crystalloids

- Normal Saline (NS), Lactated Ringers (LR)
  - Crystalloid fluid replacement ratio is 1:3 (blood loss to crystalloid fluid)

Colloids

- Hextend (6% Hetastarch in LR), Hespan (6% Hetastarch in NS), Albumin (a natural colloid)
  - Hextend is the colloid of choice in trauma

Blood Products

- Packed RBCs (PRBCs), Fresh Frozen Plasma (FFP), Cryoprecipitate (Cryo), Platelets
- A patient with a HgB <6 and HcT <18% almost always requires blood products
  - HgB >10 and HcT >30% rarely requires blood transfusion

Femoral Artery Catheterization Landmarks

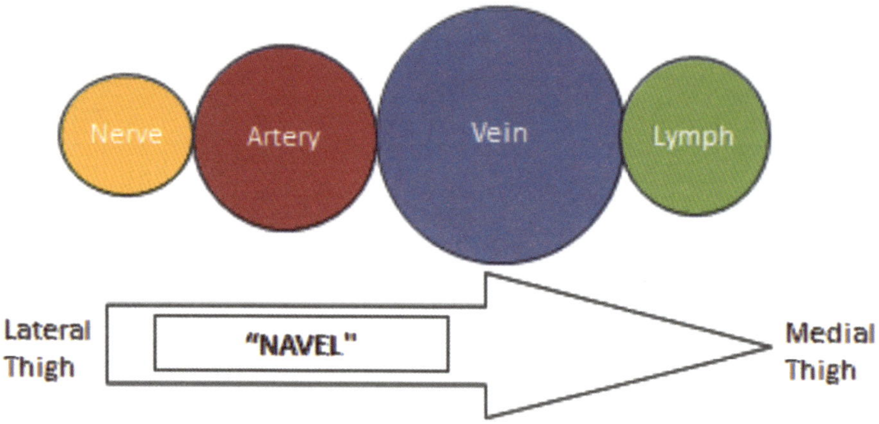

Blood Products

Packed RBCs (PRBCs)

- Made by removing 90% of the plasma and adding an anticoagulant
- Reduced risk of febrile reactions due to low plasma levels
- Transports oxygen and nutrients, contains NO clotting factors
- MUST be "Typed and Cross Matched" (ABO compatibility and Rh matching)
    - Type O negative is the universal donor for red blood cells
- 1 Unit of PRBCs will raise HgB 1g/dL and Hct 3%

Fresh Frozen Plasma (FFP)

- Plasma that has had RBCs separated
- Most useful for the clotting factors it contains (used to treat coagulopathy)
    - Has antibodies
    - Does NOT have platelets
- FFP requires ABO compatibility
    - Does not require Rh compatibility
    - Type AB positive is "universal donor" for plasma
- 1 Unit of FFP per 4 units of PRBCs

Cryoprecipitate (Cryo)

- Contains Factor VIII, von Wildebrand Factor (vWF), Fibrinogen
- In trauma it is most often used to treat Disseminated Intravascular Coagulopathy (DIC)
- Can also be used to treat Hemophilia and von Wildebrand's Dz (MC congenital bleeding abnormality)
    - Does not require ABO compatibility or Rh matched

Platelets

- Isolated from whole blood
- Used in conjunction with PRBC transfusions
  - Does not require ABO compatibility, should be Rh matched (if possible)
- Often given as a "6 Pack," 6 units over one hour.
  - 1 unit = 50ml

Blood Type	Antigen on Red Blood Cells	Antibodies in Plasma	Can Receive Blood from	Can Donate Blood to
A	A	Anti-B	A and O	A and AB
B	B	Anti-A	B and O	B and AB
AB (universal recipient)	A and B	Neither	AB, A, B, and O	AB only
O (universal donor)	Neither	Anti-A and Anti-B	O only	O, A, B, and AB

Type O Neg is universal red cell donor when there is not enough time to type and cross match

Transfusion Reactions

Stop the transfusion if there is any adverse reaction

- Drop in blood pressure
- Fever
- Tachycardia
- Pallor
- Cyanosis

Anaphylactic reaction

- Urticaria, pruritus, hypotension, tachycardia
- Caused by Anti-IgA antibodies
- Rapid onset (within 30 minutes of infusion)
- Stop the transfusion
- Epinephrine
- Steroids
- Benadryl

Overload Reaction

- Hypertension, distended neck veins
- Can occur at any time
- Stop the transfusion, administer Lasix
- More likely in those with kidney or cardiac disease

Hemolytic Reaction

- Palpitations, abdominal/back pain, syncope, "sense of doom"
- Caused by ABO incompatibility
- Slow onset (45-90 minutes)
- Stop the infusion
- Keep urine output high (100ml/hr)
- Monitor

Urticarial Reaction

- Local erythema, hives, itching
- Administer IV Benadryl
    - Administration can continue unless other adverse reactions occur

Febrile Reaction

- Fever, flushing, palpitations
- Caused by bacterial lipopolysaccharides and anti-leukocyte antibodies
- Administer IV Acetaminophen (Ofirmev™)
    - Infusion can continue if no other symptoms present

Transfusion Related Acute Lung Injury (TRALI)

- Leading cause of transfusion related death
- Patient presents with dyspnea, tachycardia, fever, cyanosis
- Caused by a reaction to leukocyte antibodies in plasma portion of blood products
- Causes acute pulmonary edema
- Symptoms begin 1 to 6 hours after transfusion
- STOP THE TRANSFUSION

Hypocalcemia (Ca <8.2 mg/dL)

- Results from the citrate found in the blood storage bags
    - DO NOT squeeze the donor blood bag (it will force excess citrate into your patient)
- Leads to hypocalcemia
- Evidenced by positive Chovstek's and Trousseaue's signs
- Administer Calcium Gluconate

2, 3 DPG (Oxygen Dissociation Curve)

- Describes how blood carries and releases oxygen.
- Relates oxygen saturation SaO_2 and partial pressure of oxygen in the blood PaO_2
- "Hemoglobin affinity for oxygen"
    - How readily hemoglobin acquires and releases oxygen molecules into the fluid that surrounds it.

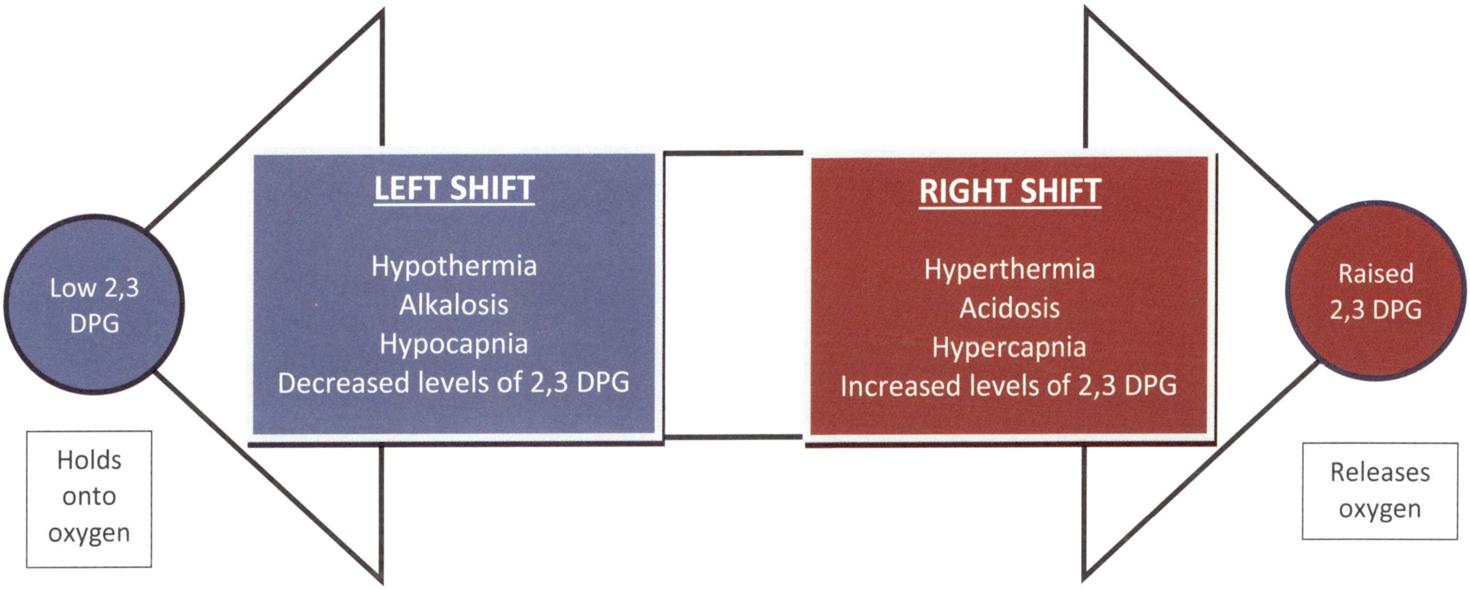

Pneumonic: CADET, face Right!" for CO_2, Acid, 2,3-DPG, Exercise and Temperature

Remember: Transfusions of blood have high citrate levels and low 2, 3 DPG levels. Thus, large transfusions can lead to hypocalcemia and lower the 2, 3 DPG levels in the body.

Quick Reference Charts

Ventilator Setting	Normal Value
Vt (Tidal Volume)	6-10cc/kg
F (Rate)	8-20/min
Ve (Minute Volume)	F x Vt (4-8 L/min)
I:E (**I**nspiratory:**E**xpiratory ratio)	1:2
FiO2 (**F**raction of **I**nspired **O**xygen)	0.21 to 1.0 (21% - 100%)
Pplat (**Pl**ateau **P**ressure)	<30
PEEP (**P**ositive **E**nd **E**xpiratory **P**ressure)	5
PEFR (**P**eak **E**xpiratory **F**low **R**ate)	500 to 700 L/min for males, 380 to 500 L/min for females

Oxygen Adjustment Calculation	(FiO2 x P1) / P2
Torr Values	
Sea Level	760 torr (1 ATM)
18k MSL	380 torr (1/2 ATM)

AMI Locations "PAILS"	EKG Leads	Vessel	Treatment
Posterior	Reciprocal changes in V1,V2,V3,V4	LCX or RCA	MONA
Anterior	V2, V3, V4	LAD	MONA
Inferior	II, III, aVF	RCA	Fluids (no nitro/ Beta Blockers)
Lateral	1, V5, V6, aVL	LCX or RCA	MONA
Septal	V1, V2	LAD	MONA

Cause	Offending Agent	Treatment
Methanol	Methyl Alcohol, Wood Alcohol, Sterno	IV Ethanol or Fomepizole
Uremia	Kidney failure	Dialysis
DKA	Diabetic Ketoacidosis	IV Fluid Resusc/Insulin
Propylene Glycol	Liquid agent used in Diazepam/Lorazepam	Flumazenil (Romazicon)
Isoniazid (INH)/Iron	Tuberculosis medication/Iron supplements	Supportive Care/Deferoxamine
Lactate	From anaerobic metabolism	Correct inadequate tissue perfusion
Ethylene Glycol	Antifreeze	IV Ethanol or Fomepizole
Salicylates	Aspirin	Dialysis

ABG	Normal Range
pH	7.35 - 7.45
CO2	35 – 45
HCO3	22 – 26
PaO2	80-100
SaO2	> 95%
Base (Excess/Deficit)	(-2) to (2+)

Chem 7 (BMP)	Normal Range
Na	135 – 145
K	3.5 – 5
Cl	95 – 105
HCO3	22 – 26
BUN	6 – 24
Cr	.7 - 1.4
Glucose	80 – 120

Medical Emergency	Treatment
Diabetic Ketoacidosis (DKA)	IV Fluids/insulin
Hyperosmolar Non-Ketotic Hyperglycemia (HHNK)	IV Fluids/insulin
Syndrome of Inappropriate Anti-Diuretic Hormone (SIADH)	Hypertonic Saline
Diabetes Insipidus (DI)	Vasopressin/DDAVP
Esophageal Varicies	Somatostatin (Sandostatin)
Mallory Weiss/Boerhaave's Tear	Supportive Care/EGD
Thyrotoxicosis/Graves's Disease	IV Fluids/ Beta Blocker/Dexamethasone/Tylenol
Hypothyroidism/Myxedema Coma	Levothyroxine (Synthroid)
Addison's Disease (Adrenal Insufficiency)	Steroids
Liver Failure	Lactulose
Septic Shock	Treat underlying cause/ Levophed
Pancreatitis	Treat underlying cause/ Demerol for pain
Hyperkalemia	Albuterol, Bicarb, Calcium Gluconate, Dextrose, Lasix, Kayexalate
Hypokalemia	Potassium

Pediatric Age Ranges	
Neonate	Birth to 28 days
Infant	28 days to one year
Toddler	One year to two years
Child	>Two Years old
Emergency Intervention Formulas	
ETT Diameter	(16 + Age)/4
	"2/3/4"
Suction/NG/Foley	**2** x ETT (i.e. 5mm ETT → 10fr Foley)
ETT insertion depth	**3** x ETT size (i.e. 5mm ETT → 15mm insertion depth)
Chest Tube	**4** x ETT (i.e. 5mm ETT → 20fr chest tube)
Normal B/P	90 + (2 x Age)
Hypotensive B/P	70 + (2 x Age)
Fluid Resuscitation (EMERGENCY)	Max of 2 bolus infusions
Neonate/Infant	10cc/kg
Toddler/Child	20cc/kg
Fluid Maintenance (NON-EMERGENT)	**"4/2/1"**
1-10 kg	**4**cc/kg/h
10-20 kg	**2**cc/kg/hr
>20 kg	**1**cc/kg/hr
Glucose Management	D-Stick <60mg/dL, All ages 2cc/kg
Neonate	D10
Infant	D25
Toddler/Child	D50

Toxic Agent	Antidote
Aspirin (ASA)	Bicarb
Benzos	Flumazenil (Romazicon)
Beta Blockers	Glucagon
Calcium Channel Blockers	Calcium Gluconate
Cocaine	Benzodiazepines
Crotalinae Snakes (Pit Vipers)	CroFab, FabAV
Cyanide	Amyl Nitrate, Sodium Nitrate, Sodium Thiosulfate
Digitalis	Digibind, Digoxin Fab
Dilantin	Supportive Care
Ethylene Glycol	IV Ethanol, Fomepizole (Antizol)
Hydrocarbons	Intubate
Isoniazid (INH)	Pyridoxine
Iron	Defroxamine
Methanol	IV Ethanol
Opiods	Naloxone (Narcan)
Organophosphates	Atropine/2-Pam Chloride
Tricyclic Antidepressants	Bicarb
Tylenol	Mucomyst/Acetadote

Fahrenheit	Celsius
105	40.6
104	40
103	39.4
102	38.9
101	38.3
100	37.8
99	37.2
98	36.7
97	36.1
96	35.6

BCCTPC
Board For Critical Care Transport Paramedic Certification®

FP-C Recertification Requirements

Immediate Action Medicine, LLC is a BCCTPC approved continuing education provider, go to our website www.immediateactionmedicine.org for course availability, services, and products. We can provide instruction anywhere around the world based on the needs of the client. Our staff is professional, experienced, and disciplined; your program will benefit from our instruction methods. We can facilitate a proctored written exam at your location or help your company coordinate online testing.

You must have 100 Continuing Education hours in critical care medicine (flight physiology, trauma medicine, toxicology, etc.) and have attended a certified recertification course (16 hours minimum). Although your certification is good for 4 years, you need to start your recertification process 6 months prior to certification expiration. Remember that CME logs are 100% audited, so don't fake your records. Things that are not acceptable for CEUs are BLS, ACLS, PALS, PHTLS, PEPP, etc. Keep good track of CEUs you take (a log is on pages 146-148). Your Training/Medical Officers can give you classes related to CEUs and you can also get credit for conference attendance. It is your responsibility to remain educated and relevant to your mission.

BCCTPC
4835 Riveredge Cove
Snellville, GA
30039
(770) 978-4400
info@bcctpc.org
www.bcctpc.org

Continuing Education (CE) Verification Log

Full Name: ____ FP-C Number:

Mailing Address:____

Email Address: ____ Phone:

Employer:

I affirm that the following information is true. (sign) ____________________________ Date:

CE Renewal

FP-C 's seeking certification renewal must accumulate 100 Contact Hours (continuing education credits) within the four-year period prior to certification expiration. At least 75 of the contact hours must be in the CLINICAL category, and up to 25 may be in the OTHER category.

Directions

Print or type all information legibly. Please refer to the CE guidelines for more information. This form may be photocopied. Submit your verification log, copies of CE documents and required fees to: BCCTPC, Attn: CE Renewal, 4835 Riveredge Cove, Snellville, GA 30039

Program Title	Date(s) of Program	Sponsoring Organization	Clinical CE's Awarded	Other CE's

.				
.				
.				
.				
14.				
		TOTAL		

Category: Publications

Name of Publication	Publish or Copyright	Type of Publication	Author or Editor	Clinical CE's Awarded	Other CE's Award
			TOTAL		

Category: Item Writing

Name of Professional Exam	Month/Year when Questions were Written	Number of Questions Written	Clinical CE's Awarded	Other CE's Awar
		TOTAL		

Category: Presentations/Lectures

Conference Name	Lecture Title	Date of Lecture	Clinical CE's Awarded	Other CE's Award

Category: Preceptorship

(Contact hours are earned only when you provide training to a student for a quarter, semester or trimester)

Name of Academic Course (provided practical training)	Month/Year	Semester, Quarter or Trimester	Number of Course Credit Hours (the student earned)	Clinical CE's Awarded	Other CE's
			TOTAL		

Category: Academia

Name of Academic Course	Month/Year	Semester, Quarter or Trimester	Total Course Credit Hrs	Grade	Clinical CE's Awarded	Other CE's
1.						
2.						
3.						

TOTAL

Total Clinical CE: ______________________________ Total Other CE_________

References

Advanced Trauma Life Support Program for Doctors: ATLS. Chicago: ACS, 2008. Print.

Bledsoe, Bryan E., and Randall W. Benner.*Critical Care Paramedic*. Upper Saddle River, NJ: Pearson Prentice Hall, 2006. Print.

Commission for the Accreditation of Medical Transport Systems Standards, 9th Edition, 2012, www.camts.org

Dubin, Dale. *Rapid Interpretation of EKG's: a New, Simplified Approach for Systematically Reading Electrocardiograms.* Tampa: Cover, 1970. Print.

Holleran, Reneé Semonin. *ASTNA Patient Transport: Principles and Practice*. St. Louis, MO: Mosby, 2010. Print.

Marx, John A., Robert S. Hockberger, Ron M. Walls, James Adams, and Peter Rosen.*Rosen's Emergency Medicine: Concepts and Clinical Practice*. Philadelphia: Mosby/Elsevier, 2010. Print.

Pierce, Graham. "Flight Paramedic Certification Testing and Renewal."*BCCTPC*. BCCTPC, 15 Jan. 2009. Web. 02 July 2011. <http://www.bcctpc.org>.

Rayman, Russell B. *Clinical Aviation Medicine*. New York, NY: Professional Pubishing Group, 2006. Print.

Reinhart, Richard O. *Basic Flight Physiology*. New York: McGraw-Hill, 2008. Print.

Tintinalli, Judith E., and J. Stephan.Stapczynski.*Tintinalli's Emergency Medicine: a Comprehensive Study Guide*. New York: McGraw-Hill, 2011. Print.

Walls, Ron M., and Michael F. Murphy.*Manual of Emergency Airway Management*. Philadelphia: Wolters Kluwer Health/Lippincott Williams & Wilkins, 2008. Print.

Images

Axillary Lines. Photograph. *Wikipedia, the Free Encyclopedia*. Web. 04 July 2011. <http://en.wikipedia.org>.

Cardiac Output Transducer. Photograph. *ISPUB - Internet Scientific Publications*. Web. 02 July 2011. <http://www.ispub.com>.

Cardiac Tamponade Chest Xray. Photograph. *BMJ Case Reports - BMJ Journals*.Web. 02 July 2011. <http://casereports.bmj.com>.

Chest X-Rays. Photograph. Wikipedia, the Free Encyclopedia. Web.15 June 2012 <http://en.wikipedia.org>.

Congestive Heart Failure Chest Xray. Photograph. Web.

Coronary Artery Diagram. Photograph. *Texas Heart Institute*. Web. 02 July 2011. <http://texasheartinstitute.org>.

Decorticate and Decerebrate Posturing. Photograph.Web. 02 July 2011. <http://hansmednotes.blogspot.com>.

Electrical Alternans EKG. Photograph. Web.

EKGs, multiple. Photograph. *Wikipedia, the Free Encyclopedia*. Web. 02 July 2011. <http://en.wikipedia.org>.

Fetal Heart Rate and Tocometry Strips. Photograph. Wikipedia, the Free Encyclopedia. Web. 02 July 2011. <http://en.wikipedia.org>.

Gastroschesis. Photograph. *Www.yoursurgery.com*. Web.

Hyperkalemia 12 Lead EKG. Photograph. Web. 02 July 2011. <http://ncbi.nlm.nih.gov>.

Hypocalcemia. Photograph. *Welcome to Best Practice*. Web. 02 July 2011. <http://bestpractice.bmj.com>.

IABP Waveforms. Photograph. *ModernMedicine - Medical Resource, Medical Information, Medical Articles*.Web. 02 July 2011. <http://modernmedicine.com>.

Intraortic Balloon Pump. Photograph. *U S Food and Drug Administration Home Page*.Web. 02 July 2011. <http://www.fda.gov>.

LeForte Fractures. Photograph. Web. 02 Aug 2012. <http://lifeinthefastlane.com>.

Mallampati Scoring. Photograph Web. 02 July 2011. <http://geemboomba.com>.

Mariceau's Maneuver. Photograph. Web. 04 July 2011. <http://ruraldoctoring.com>.

Omphacele. Photograph. *Www.cdc.gov*. Web

Pediatric Neck Xrays. Photograph. *Wikipedia, the Free Encyclopedia*. Web. 02 July 2011. <http://en.wikipedia.org>.

Phlebostatic Axis. Photograph. *Wordpressblog*. 02 July 2011. <http://rnnursementor.wordpress.com>.

Prehospital 12 Lead ECGs: Contiguous and Reciprocal Lead Charts. Photograph. *Paramedic Class Notes*. Web. 05 Aug. 2011. <http://www.rhmedicclass.com/index.php/prehospital-12-lead-ecg-contiguous-and-reciprocal-lead-charts/>.

Rule of Nines Burn Chart. Photograph. *Medical Lecture Notes Online*.Web. 02 July 2011. <http://medicalpptonline.blogspot.com>.

TCA Overdose EKG. Photograph. Web. 05 July 2011. <http://montefiore-em.com>.

Spinal Cord Injury Syndromes. Photograph. Web. 02 Aug 2012. <http://medical-dictionary.thefreedictionary.com>.

Swan-Ganz Catheter. Photograph. *Medicalexpo*.Web. 02 July 2011. <http://medicalexpo.com>.

Swan-Ganz Catheter Progression. Photograph. *Www.wikipedia.com*. Web.

Wolf-Parkinson-White EKG and picture. Photograph. Wikipedia, the Free Encyclopedia. Web. 02 March 2012. <http://en.wikipedia.org>.

Kyle Faudree is an experienced aeromedical provider with over 18 years of experience in the field of emergency medicine while serving in the United States Army. He holds certifications as an Aeromedical Physician Assistant (APA-C), Nationally Registered Paramedic (NREMT-P), and is Flight Paramedic Certified (FP-C). He has served as an Air Ambulance Flight Medic, Special Operations Flight Medic, Parachute Infantry Physician Assistant and as a Special Operations Aeromedical Physician Assistant.

Kyle developed the cutting-edge curriculum of the Immediate Action Medicine, LLC Flight Paramedic Certification course, which has a first-time pass rate well over 80% (the national average pass rate is 62%). He is credentialed as an ER PA at his local emergency department and has taught nearly 40 semester hours of undergraduate college courses in both core curriculum and technical emergency medicine. He is published in the Journal of Special Operations Medicine, and has spent over 10 years in the Special Operations Community. He has nearly four years total deployment time to both Iraq and Afghanistan as a Special Operations Flight Medic, Parachute Infantry Medical Officer, and Special Operations Aviation Medical Officer.

A portion of the proceeds from this book are donated by Immediate Action Medicine, LLC and North American Rescue, LLC to non-profit organizations that provide support to Special Operations Soldiers and their Family Members.